The Post-Polio Experience

The Post-Polio Experience

✦

Psychological Insights and Coping Strategies for Polio Survivors and Their Families

Margaret E. Backman, Ph.D.

iUniverse, Inc.

New York Lincoln Shanghai

The Post-Polio Experience
Psychological Insights and Coping Strategies for Polio Survivors and Their Families

iUniverse books may be ordered through booksellers or by contacting:

iUniverse
2021 Pine Lake Road, Suite 100
Lincoln, NE 68512
www.iuniverse.com
1-800-Authors (1-800-288-4677)

Names used in case studies and examples are fictitious and any resemblance to persons living or dead is coincidental.

ISBN-13: 978-0-595-38639-0 (pbk)
ISBN-13: 978-0-595-83020-6 (ebk)
ISBN-10: 0-595-38639-3 (pbk)
ISBN-10: 0-595-83020-X (ebk)

Printed in the United States of America

Special Thanks

To

Redjeb

For his support all along the way
and
for his help in editing this book

Contents

Social Encounters

Personal Relationships

Medical Care

Mental Health

List of Tables

Acknowledgments

I would like to take the opportunity to thank all those in the post-polio community who have shared their lives and insights with me over these many years.

Historical research for the chapter *A Breath Of Life: Psychological Reactions To The "Iron Lung"* was in part conducted at the Library of the ICD International Center for the Disabled in New York City, which at the time was under the direction of the now-retired Chief Librarian, Helen Stonehill.

INTRODUCTION

In the late 1940s through the mid 1950s poliomyelitis, a viral illness, reached epidemic proportions in the United States, as well as in other parts of the world. Most of those affected were infants and children; thus, polio became known as "infantile paralysis." Many children died, others were disabled to varying degrees. Many spent months in hospitals and convalescent homes, separated from their families and schoolmates. Some could only breathe with the help of an "iron lung." Later, patients would have intensive physical therapy and a series of operations to help them walk again. The media was filled with photos of children using crutches and wheelchairs.

Adults were not spared. In fact the President of the United States, Franklin D. Roosevelt, contracted the illness as an adult and had to use a wheelchair during his presidency. Despite the devastating potential of this virus, many of those afflicted survived with little to no weakness.

As the incidence of the disease declined because of the vaccines, polio treatment centers were closed, and the National Foundation for Infantile Paralysis focused attention on other areas, dropping the reference to infantile paralysis from its name.

Over time few physicians had experience working with polio patients, and medical students no longer learned about polio during their education and training.

Thus, decades later when polio survivors began developing new symptoms, there was a dearth of physicians who had the needed expertise to understand or treat these individuals. Since the disease no longer came readily to mind, many patients with post-polio symptoms were misdiagnosed, or the symptoms were minimized or dismissed as simple aging or hypochondriac complaints. Hopefully this is changing.

The general public to this day thinks of polio as a "non-issue." People may have heard about new cases in far-off countries, but most would be surprised to learn that there are close to 1.5 million survivors in North American today.

WHAT IS POST-POLIO SYNDROME?

Physical Symptoms

Not all who had polio were left with disabilities. Yet over time a significant portion of polio survivors, disabled or not, began experiencing new debilitating symptoms, now referred to as post-polio syndrome or PPS. Some of the most common symptoms are:

- fatigue,
- muscle weakness,
- joint and muscle pain,
- difficulty breathing, and
- intolerance to cold.

Early on some feared that the late effects of polio might be a reactivation of the poliovirus. But current thinking suggests that these symptoms are related to the years of overuse of certain muscles and the subsequent breakdown of motor neurons, as the stronger muscles work overtime to make up for their polio-weakened counterparts.

Psychological Reactions

Needless to say, these new symptoms cause much distress to those who are dealing with this potentially progressive and debilitating condition. In this regard there is a commonality with other neurological illnesses; however, post-polio differs in that the survivors had the acute illness years earlier, often in infancy, and now find themselves reliving the frightening memories, as the late effects of polio become more pronounced.

With these new physical symptoms comes a sense of unease about the uncertain future. People remember their own terrible bouts with polio and the other disabled children and adults they witnessed struggling to walk or to breathe. Feelings based on early experiences that had long been repressed now begin to surface, as people find themselves no longer able to do what they used to do. Fear, anxiety, and depression are all too common. Survivors find themselves having to face choices about using canes, crutches, and wheelchairs, when they may not have had to use these aids since the acute period or perhaps have never had to use them at all.

Terminology

In trying to be sensitive and "politically correct" in this day and age, one finds oneself stumbling over words. Sentences become awkward. For the purposes of this book and in deference to common usage, I have chosen to use certain terminology.

PPS. Refers to the late effects of polio, post-polio syndrome, or post-polio sequelae, as some prefer.

Survivors. Refers to those who had polio in the past. Some survivors have PPS and others do not; however, with age the number of survivors with PPS increases.

Significant others/Family members. Refers to the people (e.g., spouses, siblings, children, and friends) who form the supportive circle of those with PPS.

COPING WITH PPS: A PSYCHOSOCIAL GUIDE

This book, *The Post-Polio Experience,* is designed to help those experiencing the late effects of polio cope with the psychological and social changes that are becoming an ever-present part of their lives. The book also serves as a guide for families and friends, helping them understand what polio survivors are going through and providing insights into their own reactions to this often frightening and frustrating condition.

THE EARLY YEARS

1

THE GOOD OL' DAYS...OR WERE THEY?

In the 1940's and 50's when many of the polio epidemics occurred, the understanding of psychological reactions to illness was not as developed as today. Many early publications did not reflect the emotional side of patients, and the psychological needs of children in particular were not addressed.

Freudian psychology was still in its relative infancy in those days. Where it was most prevalent, such as the big cities in the US, people were more likely to blame parents for almost all problems that arose in a family. There was less understanding than today of child development and little attention to children's psychological reactions to illness.

The field of Health Psychology has only come about in the past years. At first it was strictly research based, but now includes supportive clinical help for the emotional needs of adults and children who have medical and physical problems. Although not widely practiced, the psychological needs of patients is becoming a part of the consciousness of physicians and other medical personnel and is included more and more in their training.

In the early years, the lay public usually felt it was best to keep your fears and anxieties to yourself. To show your emotions was considered a weakness, and indeed today you will still hear this view expressed, particularly by males. A dictum in the Marine Corps, so I have been told, is:

"You aren't cold unless you think you're cold."
"It doesn't hurt unless you think it hurts."

But even the military is taking a second look at these ideas, with more and more veterans having emotional problems as a result of psychological traumas suffered in times of war. Keeping your feelings repressed is not always the best way to deal with upsetting memories from the past.

Today people feel freer expressing their emotional needs and feelings. That may be positive, but a negative outcome of Freudian analysis is the blaming of parents for an array of their children's problems. There is of course a case to be made that parents exert a significant influence on their children. But other events and interactions, as well as a child's innate personality, also need to be considered in understanding their development. Parents may not be totally off the hook, but the hook that they were on in the 1950's was a pretty hefty one.

Children in earlier days were expected "to be seen and not heard."—unlike today's USA, where if a child is seen and not heard they're taken to a therapist to see what is the matter with them. But the earlier attitude in the past did not work well for the children in hospitals and convalescent homes, who in many cases learned to suffer in silence.

Some children, especially those who were about four, five, or six years old, thought that they got polio because they had been bad, that God was punishing them. They rarely told anyone of their fears. They learned that if they cried or complained, they would be considered "bad patients." Punishment and threats were one of the means that the caretakers used to exert control over their young patients. So those who were homesick, those who were scared, those who had been abused, were often afraid of confiding in the very adults who were supposed to be taking care of them.

EARLY MYTHS

It was widely thought at the time that after a short while infants and children adjusted to their hospital stay with little upset or emotional upheaval. That myth lead the caretakers to see children who were upset as "spoiled" or just looking for attention. (Indeed the looking-for-attention may have been true, but not necessarily a negative thing.)

Polio patients got the message, either directly or indirectly: They were to keep sad feelings and anxieties to themselves. Many survivors, therefore, not hearing their peers complain, felt "different" and "inadequate," as they assumed others were adjusting better than they were. So they kept silent. They did not share their worries with each other nor with their parents or the medical personnel. They rarely spoke of their polio experiences, even when they were older.

This repression has had an impact on how polio survivors cope today, as it is hard for many to speak about their fears and worries—those from the past and those in the future.

EARLY HEALTH CARE

At the height of the polio epidemics many institutions found themselves understaffed. In a lot of cases staff members, who were in direct contact with the little patients, were not well trained. Being overwhelmed with their workloads they preferred compliant patients.

But not to let this sound like a story out of Charles Dickens, many polio survivors report that they had good care, made good friends with their little fellow patients, and that their parents were always there for them. However a significant number of survivors were not so fortunate. They report unpleasant memories related to their care, enough so that decades later they are still troubled by these experiences.

Basically it was not a lack of concern, but a reflection of health care as practiced in those days and of the child-rearing practices of the time. And it was not just a lack of awareness of the needs of children, but also of the needs of families and friends in coping with the difficulties that came when polio struck a loved one.

In those years physicians were often seen as being brusque, condescending, noncommittal and indifferent. The medical culture was very hierarchical with the physician at the top, almost in a God-like position.

You still can find this highly authoritarian approach, but the interactions and communications with physicians are changing. Research has shown that open communication between doctor and patient actually leads to better health outcomes. Doctors can learn much by listening to their patients. Unfortunately in today's world, as the result of managed care, doctors are too rushed. Although they would like to listen more, they feel they cannot spare the time.

Nurses, given the nature of their work, are often closer to patients than are physicians. They know them better, and they spend more time with them giving direct care. But as in every profession there are good nurses and some not so good. This is related to both personality and training.

Decisions may be made on the basis of the convenience of the staff (who may be under-trained, overworked, and poorly supervised). Thus, the experience of making the child with polio be "normal" and "fit in", may have started in the hospitals. The "be like everyone else" would come later, when children were encouraged to "blend in" so as not to draw attention to their having had polio. These repressive practices most likely lead to a lot of the psychological conflicts that polio survivors have toward the medical profession today.

2

DEVELOPMENTAL STAGES: "I GOT POLIO WHEN I WAS..."

One of the first things polio survivors tell me is how old they were when they got polio—be it 10 months, 10 years, or whatever. Instinctively polio survivors know that age of onset is a very significant factor in:

- how they experienced the illness,
- how their families experienced the illness,
      and
- how they coped with life afterwards.

With this in mind, let us take a look at the childhood stages of development. In so doing we may better understand how the child perceived the polio experience, and how this would influence his or her personality and later adjustments to life.

CHILDREN'S REACTION TO ILLNESS

Infancy and Early Childhood

When polio occurred at the preverbal stage of development, the little patients did not have the vocabulary to help them express their feelings and needs. Because infants were not able to communicate and had no outlet for their feelings, except perhaps crying, early experiences remained in the unconscious. The lack of verbal labels attached to their emotions meant that painful and frightening events associated with medical procedures, physical restraints, and ventilators, were not consciously remembered later on.

The underlying feelings, however, could still surface at a later date, triggered by something that stirred the memory. But without the verbal cues, the person can become bewildered by the emerging feelings that seem to come from nowhere. In later years, many of those who had polio in infancy or early childhood may experience isolated symptoms, such as free-floating anxiety or shortness of breath in stressful situations. Without psychotherapy to help them make the verbal connections, they may not realize why they are experiencing these feelings and may find themselves in a state of panic, thinking that something is wrong with them mentally.

In the days before the polio vaccines, it was not the custom to have parents visit on a regular basis, let alone sleep overnight in the hospital room. In fact the little patients were often in quarantine, with very limited contact with familiar faces, if at all.

There is some thought that children can tolerate short separations from their mothers or primary caretakers up to 9 months of age. But the impact of these separations is not well understood.

Preschool: Ages 1–3 Years

During the first two years of life, children are still very dependent upon their parents and cannot understand why the parents are not able to make their pain and discomfort go away. Young children may blame their parents for causing their disease.

The initial emotional reaction is anger, often expressed as demanding and clinging behavior. If the caretakers (parents and/or nurses and doctors) do not understand the reason for this behavior and react harshly, the child can feel rejected and withdraw in despair.

Separation anxiety. Children with polio also could not understand why their parents did not save them from the doctors and the hospitals and convalescent homes. And of course they did not understand why their parents were not there with them, protecting them and taking care of them.

Separation from parents at this early age can have a severe effect on later emotional development, resulting in separation anxiety and dependency. The children feel that the absent parents have abandoned them. Anxiety and depression set in as the little patients begin to fear that they can no longer depend upon their parents, or that they may never see their parents again.

In today's thinking, a parent or a supportive other should be included as much as possible in the medical visits and hospitalizations, particularly after about 9 months. But this was not always done in years past. Fear of separation from the primary caretakers (usually the mother) peaks at about age 3 and gradually declines after that to age 6 or 7, when youngsters can better understand what is going on—not to say that they don't miss their parents, but that they can tolerate such separation better.

Lack of trust. Some children who had polio were not informed about the hospitalization, only to find themselves suddenly taken away from their parents and put in a strange environment, where they may have been physically restrained, stuck with needles, put in an iron lung, or had other unpleasant treatments.

Their language was not yet developed to the point that one could readily communicate with these young children. So when older, many had trace memories and disturbing feelings related to these early experiences that they could not understand.

To stop the young patients from crying, adults often fell back on "white lies," such as telling them that they would be going home sooner than actually was to be the case. This set the stage for distrust of authority, which can last into adulthood. Trust is important and adults should not promise anything they cannot deliver, but they often did. It is in these young years that the basis of trust and mistrust is laid down.

Today children are given better preparation when going to see a doctor or when going to the hospital. In keeping with their age, they are told what to expect as a way of alleviating anxiety, and parents are included as supportive figures more than in the past.

Lack of mobility. In addition, children between 1 and 3 years of age are very active. They do not accept physical restraint easily. Lack of mobility, plus the restrictions of hospitalization, can be particularly hard on them.

Shame and doubt. Early childhood is the period where children struggle with issues of shame and doubt, and develop their sense of autonomy. Toilet training, which normally takes place during this stage, plays a significant role in the developmental struggle. The child with polio may have had problems with toilet training as a result of the illness, but the involvement of others besides the mother cannot be overlooked.

Whether those in the medical facilities were patient and helpful enough in encouraging these children cannot always be known. But this is the period where the children learn about control and begin to form a self-image and pride. If they were called bad or punished for lack of control or cooperation during this time, their personality development may have been negatively affected. Some of these early traumas can be overcome later, but an accumulation of these negative effects can take its toll.

Ages 3–6 Years

Theoretically, since children, three and older, have more mature verbal and cognitive functioning, their patterns of psychological adjustment to illness would be more complex, as contrasted to the isolated symptoms infants develop. Later in life, these psychological reactions might appear as unresolved issues of dependency, submission, and helplessness.

After age 3, children have more awareness of themselves and their environment, including more awareness of their body parts and functions. This also leaves them vulnerable to fears of physical assault. During these years, they also begin to communicate more coherently, but with language comes the development of fearful fantasies. Understanding of reality is not well developed: Even seeing another child needing assistance for breathing, for example, can be terrifying. They may falsely interpret this as a punishment the other child is getting for being bad.

An interaction of psychological development and early hospital experiences is illustrated by the reactions of Jim, who still becomes quite anxious even when going to the doctor.

Jim was almost six years old when he was hospitalized. It was the first time he had been separated from his mother. He said he found the hospital very institutional, cold, unattractive and frightening. He actually shuddered when telling me. Jim remembers not liking the nurses. He said he particularly hated the thermometer. When asked if it was a rectal thermometer, he replied, "Yes, and I felt violated and exposed."

On the same theme, he said that he also hated the hospital gown—that he felt "naked underneath, vulnerable. People could see your body. It was the same with the thermometer. I was always a very private person," he would explain.

Jim also remembers when he was wheeled into the operating room, screaming and crying. "I felt like I would never come back. I wasn't afraid of dying," he explained. "I didn't know where I was going, and I was afraid I would be separated from my parents, particularly my mother."

Jim's experience illustrates his early fears of separation, as well as his feelings of vulnerability. Jim's extreme modesty and concerns about his body are typical for a child of that age; in his case, however, these feelings stayed with him into adulthood.

Children 3 to 6 years of age are beset by fantasies and often fear mutilation of their bodies. Polio was certainly an assault on the body—the body image and the body integrity. Since physicians and nurses usually did not speak directly to the children, overhearing conversations amongst adults—who spoke in front of them as though they were not there—added to the terrifying fantasies and contributed to feelings of depersonalization. Perhaps this is familiar to you.

When adult patients, who have experienced such traumatic events as children, face medical care again in life, they may become extremely anxious. Physicians may not understand the underlying cause of the patients' anxieties and may become impatient with the constant questioning or misinterpret the patients' behaviors.

School-Age: 7–12 Years Old

For early school-age children, understanding is at a fairly concrete level. They tend to latch onto simple and often erroneous explanations for illness, such as attributing it on something they ate or having fallen into a mud puddle. Often their emotional responses fluctuate between being angry at significant others, such as their parents or the doctors and nurses, to self-blame.

With moral development comes the development of a conscience, and at this concrete stage of understanding children may blame themselves for their illness or, as with the younger children, interpret illness as a punishment for being bad. As a way of coping, some polio patients learned to be the "good patient," that is compliant and not making waves.

As children get older, their understanding of reality develops more fully, and they deal with anxiety through intellectualization, i.e. mental reasoning rather than emotions. During this period of development, the child has a need for information that is clear, relevant, and realistic. Concrete explanations begin to give way to more valid understandings of the cause of illness. More realistic understanding of what has happened and what is going on appears at this stage.

During these early school years, children may tolerate the effects of illness better than when younger or older. Although they still need adequate support and preparation, they can tolerate separation from parents better than younger children, and are less involved in the turmoil of adolescence. They can make use of intellectualization and rationalization, and their anxieties can be lessened by clear explanations of what is about to happen. Unfortunately, during the period when many had polio, children were often not informed or where misinformed, adding to their confusion and anxiety.

Understanding death. Typically, children do not comprehend the realities of death until they are about eight to ten years of age. However, children who have been seriously ill and hospitalized can come to face death at an earlier age. One does not always think about young patients thinking about death. But having seen other patients suffering and "disappearing", these secret fears are deep inside. They wonder what is going to happen to them.

Those who have had to depend upon machines to breathe may realize much earlier the possibility of their own death—even before they are psychologically ready to handle this. Thus, the fear of death becomes a reality that can get repressed with other frightening memories.

Puberty and Adolescence

By the beginning of puberty, a child's emotional reactions become even more complex. The question "Why me?" begins to be heard. At this stage children may feel sorry for themselves and brood for days. Philosophical and religious explanations may be used to help them deal with illness.

The struggle for identity marks adolescence and group acceptance and recognition becomes important (Erickson, 1959). When adolescents become ill, feelings of inadequacy and of not being a complete person can dominate their thoughts. Self-esteem, which is shaped by peer reinforcement, suffers. Some teens carry denial to an extreme and act in ways that are actually detrimental to their health, i.e., drinking alcohol when contraindicated by medication, or engaging in strenuous sports when told not too. This pattern can continue throughout life.

Although the cosmetic implications of an illness are important at all ages, they are of considerable significance in adolescence, when appearance, identity, and acceptance become of prime concern. Disfigurement and disability may affect self-image. How these problems are handled depends in part upon the reactions of others.

For the adolescent, lack of control and dependency can be particularly devastating. This is a stage when young people learn to separate from their parents and take control of their lives and bodies.

When afflicted with polio in the adolescent years, the young person may have become more dependent on, and demanding of, peers, friends and family; or they may have withdrawn and been moody for months.

Some young patients reacted to their lack of freedom, as it felt to them, by acting out, or "being bad." Behind this was a way to draw attention to themselves. But acting out is often not what it appears to be on the surface.

A Case of Sexual Abuse

In one case, a polio survivor told me that she had been repeatedly sexually abused by a physical therapist during what was to be her PT treatment. She was afraid to tell anyone, as the therapist had threatened her. But her protestations about not wanting to go to therapy were only met by the insistence of the staff. Finally she started hiding on the grounds of the convalescent home, only to be found and punished. She was not being a "good patient."

Later, as an adult, she would find out that her chart had labeled her a difficult patient, something which today makes her feel very angry and further reinforced her distrust of authority.

Also, her sexual trauma had never been dealt with. In fact it took quite some time for her as an adult in psychotherapy to even breach the subject. It was a secret she kept all her life, telling no one including her husband.

To this day, little is known about the part that abuse played in the polio experience. Physical and sexual abuse was not talked about as openly as today, and children often feared not being believed, and they were probably right in most cases.

GOING HOME

Hospitalization was difficult, but on the positive side the young polio patients were in a community of youngsters their own age who had similar problems. Many of these polio patients made life-long friendships that lasted throughout their lives.

Going home, however, did not come without anxieties. How would they fit in? Would people think they were contagious? How would they manage being on a respirator? What if they had problems walking?

Children in hospitals and convalescent homes often did not have regular schooling and fell behind academically and socially. In some cases young people were taken out of school and taught at home, thus missing out on important lessons in social interaction.

Those who returned to school found it difficult and embarrassing; they no longer fit in. Issues surfaced with schoolwork and personal habits. Having spent so much time with adults in the hospitals and respiratory centers, these children revealed a maturity that others their age did not have and could not understand. Yet many were socially awkward, alternating between mature and immature behavior.

For adolescents who had polio it was particularly difficult. Many were teased or ostracized and discriminated against in obvious and subtle ways. Some faced restrictions on their physical activity and athletic participation, limiting their chances to find an outlet for their energies or to find an identity in school. What the school administrators and teachers saw was rebellious acting-out, or the contrary, shyness, over-dependency, or unexplained anger.

Unfortunately for many, treatment did not end upon returning home. Periodic hospitalizations for surgery or other interventions took the young person out of school for varying periods of time—further compromising academic performance and socialization.

Some whose schooling was interrupted by polio did not complete high school or college. Later in life they would feel a shame for their lack of credentials and degrees, something they would try to hide.

PSYCHOLOGICAL ISSUES

3

PSYCHOLOGICAL REACTIONS TO POLIO AND PPS

Many of the psychological issues polio survivors face are similar to those faced by others with disabilities. However, with the advent of post-polio syndrome (PPS), the weakness, the pain, and the fear of not being able to walk are reminders of the earlier episode, causing the survivor to relive overwhelming emotional feelings that had been repressed for years. As these new physical symptoms emerge, psychological issues with ties to the past begin to surface.

INTERACTION OF PERSONALITY AND ILLNESS

To understand what post-polio survivors may be going through emotionally it is important to understand how they reacted psychologically when they first contracted the disease.

Patients' underlying personalities played important roles in the way they reacted to the initial bout with polio and now to PPS. Those who had a fear of failure, for example, would be devastated by the inability to take care of themselves and would become particularly concerned about the future. Those subject to depression would become more depressed. Those with obsessive-compulsive personalities would be concerned with every detail of their care and their bodily functions in an attempt to gain some kind of control. Those already struggling with issues of dependency would be particularly upset when becoming dependent upon a ventilator.

DEFENSE MECHANISMS

People bring to a situation their own unique set of psychological defenses to protect them from distressing feelings. Under stress the defenses may begin to break down, leaving the person overwhelmed and unable to cope

A distinction is often made between coping strategies and defense mechanisms. Both are protective of the individual and both provide some satisfaction for needs.

Coping responses, however, are flexible and adaptive. They are more under conscious control and are considered more effective.

Defenses, on the other hand, are more rigid patterns of behavior that ultimately may be maladaptive. They usually operate automatically without conscious awareness and allow you to continue functioning, although in a more limited and inflexible way.

However, not all defenses are bad. It is only when they become rigid and interfere with your life that they are considered maladaptive. We need defenses to help us get through the day, so that we do no focus constantly and unnecessarily on unpleasant memories or fears.

Repression and Weakened Defenses

For years, repressed feelings and associated memories of the polio experience had been kept in check by the psychological defenses of denial, avoidance, and isolation. For many, these defenses worked well, helping the individual to go on with life. Yet many of these repressed memories and fears from childhood remained unexpressed and distorted in the unconscious. Now, however, under the stress of PPS (or other illnesses or life events) the defenses begin to break down, and the repressed feelings rise to the surface, overwhelming the individual.

The fact that someone has gone through something before is no reason to assume that it will be easier the second time around, or that the person will have a better understanding of the situation. On the contrary, having to relive the experience—an experience that the individual thought had been put to rest—reawakens anxieties and conflicts that he or she had been able to ignore for many years. As one patient explained, *"I thought I had all this behind me; I don't know if I can go through it again."*

Regressive Behavior

As most polio survivors were children or adolescents when they struggled with the disease and its aftermath, clinical observation suggests that many of the needs and behaviors that appear under the new stressful situation are reflective of childhood issues—a reliving of an earlier event.

Returning to the use of a brace or wheelchair after having struggled to overcome the need for such aids years before may activate long-standing emotional conflicts. Many of the conflicts center around issues of dependency, sometimes presenting as angry outbursts at those the patient is close to and whose help is now most needed. Fears reemerge—of being restricted and trapped, of being abandoned, fears emanating from the previous experience in hospitals and convalescent homes.

A busy physician may treat the emerging regressive behavior as an irritation. Yet such behavior is not unexpected, and may be an attempt to regain equilibrium. Not only are the defenses not working in such cases, but also many of the psychological issues are those that the survivor had dealt with as a child. What the family, physicians and rehabilitation personnel see are behaviors and ideation that, on the surface, appear excessive or unrealistic, but are in effect symptoms of the underlying emotional concerns, which cannot find appropriate release.

Patients' complaints about not being able to dance, swim, bicycle, or walk for any length of time may seem self indulgent or unrealistic to others. "After all," some may respond, "it is little to give up, if these restrictions slow down the deteriorating process." But what needs to be understood is that these *"complaints"* are expressions of fear of what is to come: fear of not being able to walk or breathe.

Complaints about not being able to drive, for example, may be expressions of anxiety related to dependency and lack of control in one's life. Resistance to wearing a leg brace may on the surface appear unrealistic, if such support is needed. But this resistance may be an expression of the person's fear of impending lack of mobility. Others may brush cosmetic complaints aside as pure vanity, but vanity is often an expression of self-esteem—an important element for successful outcomes, both physical and mental.

Avoidance and Social Withdrawal

Many of those trying to cope with the late effects of polio distance themselves from family and friends. Although going out and being with others may seem therapeutic, for some being with others may increase feelings of uncertainty, anxiety, and self-consciousness. Having been the focus of so much scrutiny during the first bout with polio, many now feel panic when anticipating social situations.

For one, they are conscious of people looking at them. Well-meaning questions or offers of help add to the self-consciousness. And the many questions that people ask often do not have ready answers. They simply serve to remind survivors that they do not know what is going to happen to them in the long run. Thus, although social interactions can be supportive, they can also be anxiety producing.

Friends, in turn, sensing the polio survivor's mood, are unsure of what to say or do. In becoming more aware of the survivor's disability, they come to face their own feelings of vulnerability and mortality.

The uneasiness of others and the polio survivor's own discomfort tend to feed upon each other, making some with PPS choose social isolation as a way of coping. Yet, in this isolation, the person with PPS is prone to focus on the negatives of his or her state, with the risk of sinking further into depression.

Denial

Denial, the psychological inability to accept what has occurred, is a very common defense where physical illness and disability are concerned. Although intellectually a person may know what has happened, the seriousness or the implications are ignored or minimized. Denial may show itself as numbness, a removal of material from consciousness, and avoidance of reminders of the condition. It can take the form of consciously or unconsciously refusing to accept new limitations imposed upon one: For example, a cardiac patient begins to smoke heavily again; a person diagnosed with post-polio syndrome undertakes strenuous risk-taking exercises and activities.

Research suggests that denial may be helpful during the early phase of a critical illness but later on can exact a price. Early on, denial gives the person the time needed to adjust to the shock of what is happening. However, over time the person in denial may not seek out appropriate help, may not follow medical directives, or may do things that could lead to further complications.

The need to get some relief from a chronic condition and its treatment is one of the reasons that people

a) Deny or under-react to new symptoms, or

b) Do not comply with what they are told to do.

In the short run this may be an effective coping mechanism and provide a period of relief; however, in the long run such denial, if carried too far, may not serve a protective function but instead create even more complications.

Families (and even professionals) can fall into denial as well. If others have difficulty dealing with polio or the late effects of polio, they may go along with the survivor's denial or use denial to handle their own emotions.

Picking up on the other's denial and avoidance, the person with PPS can become fearful that they are in fact too fragile to deal with the realities of their condition. Or they may fear that they are at fault for having the symptoms. This is what happened to many who had polio as children. The denial that they internalized from the family left them with poor self-esteem, as well as anger and sadness that never had the opportunity to be expressed.

How and when to confront a person who is in denial with the realities of the situation is a very difficult question to answer. Research suggests that in most situations you have better physical and mental health if you talk about your emotional distress rather than staying "bottled up".

But we must bear in mind that just as people are different, there are different stages in the adjustment to medical and psychological problems. One approach does not fit all. When confronted inappropriately or when not ready to talk or give up the denial, people simply withdraw or put up even stronger defenses.

DISTRUST OF AUTHORITY

The capacity to trust in others is laid down early in life. The lies and evasions from adults (medical personnel and parents) added to the mistrust of authority that many polio survivors have to this day.

Much of the conflict in dealing with the medical establishment revolves around earlier experiences in hospitals and convalescent homes. Patients were often not dealt with directly; they were allowed to live with their fantasies of what was happening or what would happen to them. As discussed in the chapter on developmental stages, a lack of trust developed when patients were told they would not be in the hospital for long, only to find themselves "trapped" in the hospital or convalescent home for six months or a year.

Today polio survivors question the treatment and advice they received those years ago. Some feel that the physicians did not really know what to do, and the treatment, especially the urging to do more and more, may have contributed to the PPS they have today. Thus, the not wanting to go to doctors and the questioning of medical advice is but a symptom of this mistrust of authority: *"If they didn't know what they were doing then, how do I know they know what they are doing today?"*

ANGER AND NEED FOR CONTROL

People search for meaning to explain life events. They try to apply logic or reason as a means of re-establishing control over a situation that seems out of their control. They look for a cause on a physical, emotional or spiritual level. Sometimes anger surfaces as a result of this search leading to:

- self-blame and
- blaming others, such as a doctor, a spouse, or parents.

One reason self-blame may be prevalent is that polio often struck during childhood, a developmental period when you are likely to blame things on yourself. A child does not have a global picture but lives in a rather constricted universe. At certain ages, when any problems happen in the family, a child may feel that he did something wrong or was bad and that is why this or that happened. It is a way of trying to understand the world.

Unfortunately adults or siblings may reinforce the self-blame by laying guilt on the child. Sometimes, for example, telling a child he is bad is done out of frustration and anger, or as a way of controlling a child. But this kind of interaction can leave dark deep scars.

For polio survivors, anger may be directed at their fate, at themselves for not having followed medial advice, at parents for not having helped them enough, at family for not understanding their plight, at friends for the pressure their very presence imposes.

The medical staff often takes the blunt of anger, being blamed for not caring enough, not listening, not knowing, not doing enough, letting the patient get worse and not being able to promise a cure.

Frustrations are taken out on family members and anyone else who happens to be around when the rage lets loose. Although in calmer moments one may realize that the anger is not always rational; it is a rage that comes from not having control over what has happened or is happening.

And family members too may become angry, directing some of this frustration onto the survivor, who may be blamed for not having taken care of himself, for being a burden, or for deserting the family. Survivors may be made to feel that they have caused their own symptoms by having lead a stressful life or having done too much. This reaction is now more common given the current thought that one can affect one's health by good living and a positive attitude

One never knows, perhaps some survivors contributed to their problems, or perhaps the problems would have come anyway. However, making people feel responsible for their conditions only adds to the burdens they already carry. In addition to the physical suffering, people should not have to bear the emotional suffering that comes with self-blame.

GUILT

Guilt may emerge over the anger felt toward loved ones or over feelings that others' problems have resulted from the polio, either directly or indirectly.

For example, a patient confided that she thought her son's learning disabilities had something to do with her having had polio, that somehow he had inherited this from her. Thus, there was never enough that she could do for him.

Others have expressed concern that they were not able to be as good a parent as they might have been had they been able bodied.

Still others have felt guilty for having had polio in the first place. They feel guilty for all the help they have received over the years and what they perceive as the burden they placed on the family. With guilt comes a feeling of grief, anticipatory mourning and chronic sorrow.

Guilt can stop you in your tracks. You don't know which way to move. If you feel selfish or self-centered you may feel guilty, so you neglect yourself and your needs. If you are made to feel blame, or if you are the type to blame yourself, the guilt can lead to behaviors that are not always healthy.

Significant others too may feel guilty. They feel bad about their own anger, and they often need permission from you to allow them to express this anger, frustration and guilt.

DEPRESSION AND SADNESS

If you find that you are seeing everything as black, then you may be very depressed. Nothing feels that it will work out. Anything anyone suggests to you feels useless. Why try? You don't even have the energy even if you wanted to.

Many people who have PPS say they are more depressed now than before they had polio. Men often show their depression by being angry and irritable; women are more likely to speak of sadness and crying. In many cases this is not a deep depression, but an underlying sense of sadness that does not go away. As one woman confided to me, *"I'm tired of crying; yet when not crying, it feels like I am sobbing internally."*

As the PPS symptoms get worse, the depression expresses itself as a lack of interest in life, a lack of hope. As one woman said: *"Happiness seems short-lived."*

It is not surprising then that those with PPS may have an underlying sadness and even feel quite depressed at times. Depression and sadness are normal reactions when a person's level of functioning is decreasing.

Depressive Symptoms

Poor concentration, sleep disturbance, and decreased interest in activities that you used to enjoy may be symptomatic of a depressed state. Other characteristics to look out for are described in the table Depression Signs and Symptoms that appears at the end of this chapter.

The changes that you need to make with PPS and the new health regimes that come into play can be depressing, particularly at first. Yet the depression interacts with these changes making it harder for you to manage these changes and new regimes.

Depression can make pain feel worse. It also can prevent you from going for needed help and making necessary changes in your life.

Depression seems to put a gray cloud over everything. It is as though nothing is going right or ever will. It alters your self-perception and interferes with your relationships. You may have an irritable and angry mood, you feel down all the time. People avoid you: They see you as a downer and a complainer, who seems to do nothing to help yourself. It becomes a vicious circle.

Talking of Suicide

Suicidal ideation, one of the symptoms of depression, is often a reflection of the person's sense of helplessness that comes with the uncertainty about the future. If you or someone you know appears to be suicidal, it is important to consult a psychiatrist or other physician as soon as possible. Go to a hospital outpatient clinic, if necessary.

However, in many cases the expressions of wishing to die are expressions of a deep sense of despair and do not mean that the person is really planning to take his or her life.

Often people who speak of suicide will not attempt to kill themselves, but they want to believe that they could do so if things got any worse. It is for some the last bit of control they feel that they have in their life, a way out.

Beating Depression

Psychological treatment of the depression may decrease suffering even if many of the physical symptoms of PPS still persist. The polio survivor may have developed coping mechanisms that are no longer suitable. Avoidance and denial may now serve to exacerbate problems that need attention.

In treating depression, professionals try to help patients see that they do have other options, as a way of dealing with the hopelessness. Antidepressant medication can help get someone through a difficult period. It can lift the depression enough to let the person then be able to talk through feelings and problems in psychotherapy. Some depression is related to a chemical imbalance, and in such cases a person may need to take the medication for an extended period of time. Thus, as each person is different it is important to get a good professional evaluation.

Table 1

DEPRESSION: SIGNS AND SYMPTOMS

PHYSICAL
- Lack of energy
- Trouble sleeping
- Change in appetite or weight (up or down)
- Unexplained backaches or headaches
- Stomach-aches or indigestion

MENTAL
- Difficulty concentrating
- Poor memory
- General slowing of thoughts

EMOTIONAL
- Irritability or anger
- Feelings of
    Hopelessness
    Helplessness
    Guilt—feeing like a burden to others
- Feeling empty
- Loss of interest in social activities
- Loss of sexual desire

Table 2

DEPRESSION: WHAT TO DO

- See Your Healthcare Provider:
  Have a complete checkup.
  Discuss your symptoms—
      physical, mental, and emotional.

- Talk To Family and Friends:
  See how they can help you.

- Set Realistic Goals:
  Don't expect too much of yourself.

- Avoid Stressful Situations.

- Put Off Making Major Life Changes,
  (if possible).

- Exercise (as allowed by your doctor).

- Make Time For Enjoyable Activities.

4

ABANDONMENT: A PERVASIVE ISSUE

John got polio when he was only a year old. He was sent to the Sister Kinney Institute for 6 months and saw little of his family. Today, John does not consciously remember the experience, as he was too young to put words onto what was happening. What he shares with others who had polio at a very young age is an underlying sense of isolation and a fear of being abandoned. The feelings stayed with him into adulthood. Until he addressed these feelings with a therapist, he could not understand why he "over-reacted" to things that did not bother other people as much.

Sarah was only 8 months old when she had polio. She has been told that she was in isolation at the hospital for 10 days. Like John, she was in and out of hospitals and under medical care for years. Sarah describes an underlying anxiety that people will leave her, that she will be isolated and left alone. When under stress, she finds herself re-experiencing the sense of abandonment, often reacting inappropriately to situations as though she were that child again: frightened and angry. Today she is consumed with the fear that her husband, who is older than she, will die and thus abandon her. Although she knows intellectually that she can get along on her own and has supportive people around her, she continues to feel very insecure, as if whatever she depends on will be pulled out from under her.

FEAR OF BEING ABANDONED

Those who had polio at a very young age talk of having "emotional memories"—of feeling helpless and defenseless, of being afraid to make attachments to others for fear of rejection and abandonment. As they were often left alone without the nurturance of a close family, they did not learn how to relate to others, except perhaps to teach themselves not to make trouble and try to fit in.

But there were others who did just the opposite. They tried to draw attention to themselves, so they would not be so isolated or left alone. Karen was one of these.

Karen was only 5 years old when she contracted polio. She remembers being in the hospital initially and then again when she had her surgeries. Later when she was at the convalescent home, her parents rarely visited her. She did not understand that the home was far away and that it was difficult and costly for them to visit often.

When her parents didn't show up for what felt like a long time, Karen feared that they were ill or had died. She reacted by becoming a "trouble maker", refusing to do what she was told, bothering other children, and even trying to run away. When the nurses threatened that they would send her home if she didn't behave, she acted out even more.

Going home was what she wanted. She wanted to see her mother, her father, to find out if they were alive.

Karen worried and worried that they would never come again; that she would be left on her own. Angry and frightened she refused to speak to her parents the next time they came to visit. Karen was too young to understand their explanation of why they had not been able to come—justified as it may have been. Each time after their visit she became very frightened that she would never see them again. Today, Karen is left with an underlying fear of abandonment. In her case she goes from wanting to be invisible and left alone to making waves so others will give her the care and attention that she feels she needs.

Doing Anything to Fit In

From the fear of abandonment comes the sense of not being able to take care of oneself, of being at the mercy of others. As a result, some survivors developed coping styles that lead them to be overly accommodating, overly helpful, and overly generous—anything so others would like them and be there for them.

Paulo remembers that when he went back to grade school after being in the hospital, he did not want to use any crutches or his wheelchair. He wanted to fit in with his little playmates. Now as a grown man, Paulo says that he will do "almost anything" for people, so that they will accept him. This has caused him to by very sensitive to others' needs and reactions. As a defense, he tends to isolate himself and has become a very private person.

Feeling in the Way and Useless

Despite having grown up to be quite a successful person, Bob had incorporated the sense of being useless into his personality. He was always afraid of being rebuffed, and therefore never reached out to others, as he felt the best thing he could do was just to stay out of the way. As a result people thought of him as cold and unfriendly.

Insecurity in Relationships

Art complains that he has a hard time believing that anyone could like him. When he was growing up he felt this was because he was "a cripple"—a word that some of his schoolmates used when teasing him. Who would be there for him? Who would understand? Whom could he trust? He admits to having developed an "obnoxious personality"—being arrogant and always needing to be in control. But he now recognizes that this is a way of keeping others at bay, rejecting them before they can reject him.

As the examples above show, how you experienced the sense of abandonment depends on the interaction of many factors, such as your developmental age when you became ill, your family's reaction to your situation, your particular hospital and rehabilitation experiences. All of this was dependent upon your own personality and the various personalities that you had to deal with on a day-to-day basis.

5

LOSS AND BEREAVEMENT

LOSS AND THE SENSE OF SELF

Over the years we are forced to deal with loss in one way or another. As a child it may have been the loss of a friend who moved away or the death of a pet. The death of a loved one is one of the most significant losses you may have to deal with in life.

For some people the changes in their body over time feel like a loss. The pretty unwrinkled face no longer looks out at you in the mirror:

Who is that old woman with all those lines?

The disbelief and shock from a photo:

That baldheaded man with that large belly, certainly not me.

Although these changes in appearance may not seem as serious as the loss of a person in your life, they can still have profound effects on the person involved.

If you have post-polio syndrome (PPS), there is the loss of function and what goes with that:

- Not being able to do what you used to do,
- Becoming more dependent upon others,
- Facing a change in your self-confidence and self-concept.

You may be afraid to speak about your grief and sense of loss, because when you look at others whom you see as worse off, you feel that you have no right to complain. Comparing yourself to others may help, if you feel it gives you some perspective. But don't let that make you feel that you should repress you own feelings.

What counts is how something is experienced psychologically. If you hurt, it is your hurt no matter how big or how small.

DEALING WITH LOSS AND GRIEF

Those with polio may have experienced losses as a child. Some were too young to realize what had happened. Others were so focused on improving their health and function, that they never took the time or were allowed to take the time to grieve the loss. Now that PPS is coming to the fore, the unresolved grief begins to resurface.

For the older children and adults back then, the "stiff upper lip" was reinforced as the way to survive the ordeal—the stoic approach of not showing your emotions and not complaining or dwelling on the negative.

There is something to be said for "toughing it out", but only to a degree. If you bury your grief and sorrow for too long and do not try to work it through, it can stay under the surface as a sadness and anxiety your whole life, causing you to act and react in ways that you may not like and that you cannot understand.

To cope psychologically with loss you need to be able to grieve. This means allowing yourself to recognize that a loss has occurred and to try to work through the emotional pain. What we mean by "working through" is to become aware of feelings that are related to the loss, be they sadness, guilt, anger, anxiety. Then try to channel these emotions in ways that allow you to manage them, and not have the feelings control you and take over your life in a negative way.

This is not to say that once worked through you will not have the sadness or other emotions, but you will understand them and be able to adjust and go on with your life.

For a further discussion of loss and grief from the perspective of a psychologist and polio survivor, I refer you to the insightful article (1996) by the late Jack Genskow, Ph.D. that is referenced at the end of this book.

STAGES OF ADJUSTMENT

As the symptoms of PPS progress, survivors go through an adjustment process that is similar to that of the dying: Denial, Despair, Negotiation, and Acceptance.

Denial encompasses the period of shock, of disbelief; there is an inability to face the reality of what is happening. One feels like an outsider looking in. Emotions are cut off, isolated from what is happening all around. There is the sense: "This can't be happening to me."

Following the initial shock comes *despair*. Here there is a conscious recognition that indeed this is happening to you. Feelings of anger alternating with hopelessness and deep depression appear, often affecting eating and sleeping.

Survivors report feeling emotionally flooded with disturbing and persistent thoughts of what would be: Thoughts of self, family, friends, job, upcoming treatments, and the possible prognosis. The future can appear bleak, as if there is no way out. It is during such a period that ideas about suicide may begin to emerge.

The next stage, *negotiation*, represents an attempt, feeble at first to take control, to see if perhaps all was not as bad as first thought. Doctors are questioned regarding possible alternatives. Bargaining takes place for procedures or aids that would be less uncomfortable, less cumbersome, less costly. Agreeing to cooperate and participate in treatment is often the first step toward acceptance.

What is called the period of *acceptance*, is when you intellectually and emotionally attempt to recognize the condition and its limitations, and turn your energies to problems that appear to be manageable. In coming to this state you may need to abandon some old ways of doing things and to develop new skills and interests. Basically, the stage of acceptance requires a redefinition of oneself, coupled with the discovery of positive feelings about who you are.

This adjustment process involves a search for meaning in the experience and an attempt to regain mastery over stressful life events. People do not necessarily go through these stages in sequence and may revisit them, as their situation changes.

BEREAVEMENT PROCESS

Physical losses are experienced as a symbolic or actual death of part of the body. For polio survivors the recurrence of symptoms may thrust them into the bereavement process, only to recover again, and then to go through process over and over, as additional losses appear over time.

The bereavement process for polio survivors is intensified by the reemergence of the memories and feelings long repressed. *Anger and guilt* are common emotions that come to the fore during bereavement; however, survivors may feel confused by these emotions, assuming that the issues affecting them were dealt with long ago.

6

A BREATH OF L[
PSYCHOLOGICAL REAC I IONS
TO THE "IRON LUNG"

The acute phase of polio left many patients feeling helpless, confused, and panicky. Some emerged from the upheaval only to find themselves dependent upon a mechanical aid for respiration, and often completely quadriplegic.

One of the complications of poliomyelitis was acute respiratory failure. Many patients needed either full-time or part-time mechanical ventilation (i.e. assisted breathing) for months or years, due to chronic breathing problems. Today some still rely on ventilators for survival. The more fortunate suffered no breathing difficulties and were left with little or no residual effects from the disease.

With the advent of post-polio syndrome (PPS), however, increasing numbers of former patients are finding that they are now developing respiratory problems, some for the first time. Even if they never had such problems before, many survivors have vivid memories of others who did and are fearful of what lies ahead.

STED VENTILATION DURING
HE POLIO EPIDEMICS

In the 1950's the United States was not as advanced as Britain, Scandinavia, and some other countries in the use of ventilation devices. European countries established respiratory centers, using various techniques for mechanically assisted respiration, in reaction to a major outbreak of poliomyelitis in Copenhagen, Denmark, in 1952.

Although mechanical ventilation was still in its infancy in the US, during the polio epidemics of the 1950s, Bower and his associates in Los Angeles lowered the mortality rate for those with bulbar-type polio from 90 percent to 20 percent, using a combination of techniques based on "the Drinker iron lung, tracheotomy, Bennett's extra-pressure device, and high humidity" (Dobkin, 1972, p. 78).

During that period, the National Foundation for Infantile Paralysis organized respirator centers in various parts of the United States, which relied mainly on the tank respirator. It was not until the mid-1950s that research in the United States began developing ventilators for long-term respiratory care. There has been great progress since then, especially with the introduction of portable ventilators.

Also, the eventual development of the Salk and Sabin vaccines and the mass inoculations that followed led to the eradication of polio in most of the world. However, many former patients still rely on ventilators. Fortunately, the techniques available, including portable ventilators, are more sophisticated and less restrictive than those available 50 years ago.

THE THREAT OF DEATH

When the muscles controlling respiration are paralyzed, the inability to breathe and the feeling that you are going to suffocate make the possibility of death very real. The fear of death was so overwhelming that patients handled it through massive repression—repression so extensive that it pushed unwanted memories from the conscious memory, taking with it associated thoughts and feelings, as well.

Most polio deaths were from paralysis of the patients' respiratory area. However, after the acute phase of polio, death by asphyxiation was rare. Nevertheless, the fear of dying remained in patients' minds, revealed by worries that the respiratory equipment would suffer mechanical or electrical failure.

Psychological concerns with asphyxiation are particularly associated with the mask, which was sometimes used to assist in ventilation. The mask was used, for example, when a patient was being moved and was temporarily out of the "iron lung." Now, later in life, these polio survivors might experience panic attacks when their faces are covered or when they develop shortness of breath.

THE PSYCHOLOGICAL MEANING OF THE RESPIRATOR

Ventilation devices gave patients "the breath of life", according to H. E. Van Riper, the Medical Director for the National Foundation of Infantile Paralysis in the 1950's. He reported seeing patients in iron lungs who had "almost forgotten how to breathe for themselves"—a condition which often continued long after the muscles were capable of providing adequate ventilation of the lungs (1956, p. 45).

The respirator became very important to polio patients, since it saved their lives. Patients developed different attachments to the machines, which were loved and hated at the same time. The tank respirator offered a sense of security. It became a substitute body or "a womblike structure which the patient feared to leave" (Glud & Blane, 1956).

The psychological attachment made it harder for patients to be weaned from the respirator, particularly since their bodies were so changed, having become weak and barely functional. Yet there was a conflict. Although the respirator provided life and breath, patients hated the dependency and loss of control that the machine signified.

As a result of this dependent state, many patients returned home lacking in confidence and experiencing difficulty with the ordinary activities of daily living. Over time, through the step-by-step process of rehabilitation and encouragement from family and friends, patients gradually regained both the physical and psychological strength to move ahead.

PSYCHOSOCIAL DEPRIVATION AND "THE IRON LUNG"

Psychological deprivation was associated with respirators, particularly the tank respirator or "iron lung". Patients could not be stroked or held, and the comfort that comes from touching was, therefore, limited (Report of the Surgeon General's Workshop, 1982).

When in the tank respirator, patients reported a sense of being an "island unto themselves" with little communication. If they had a dome over their heads while in the respirator, it was difficult to be heard, cutting them off even more from others and their immediate environment. Another serious restriction was the loss of the use of their hands, making it difficult or impossible to feed or dress themselves, or to communicate with others, either in writing or by expressive gestures. To cope with these deprivations, patients learned to use other people as extensions of themselves.

An overhead mirror used with tank respirators helped patients to see beyond their limited environment. However, when they saw people via the mirror, they only could see portions of peoples' bodies and portions of the area beyond. Thus, not only was self-perception fragmented, but the perceptions of others and the outside world was disjointed.

Not only did patients with polio have to contend with paralysis, but being dependent upon a ventilator severely limited their mobility as well. Such limitations are hard at any age, but for young growing patients, it was particularly difficult. Youthful energy was stifled. Movement is one way individuals discharge energy and tension. When movement is thwarted, frustration ensues.

In addition, the lack of mobility made it difficult if not impossible for these patients to take care of their oral, genital, and excretory needs. At a very deep level they felt denied their humanity, as they could not take care of these very basic matters. Thus, they felt shame, embarrassment, and anger at their dependency.

Patients on ventilators often spent months in the hospital, not knowing the difference between night and day. Only hospital rituals helped to keep them organized and aware. Since a stable environment signifies security, small changes in a patient's environment, such as a change in the position of the bed or a change of roommates, could be disturbing and take on enormous significance.

SELF-IMAGE AND INTEGRITY

By "self-image" we refer to the picture of our self and our body that we have in our mind. The picture begins to form by nine months of age and develops over time. It is representative of the present and the past, and changes as the individual learns new skills and has new experiences.

For those in an "iron lung," self-image was challenged on a very basic level. Researchers in the 1950's reported that polio patients become overly concerned with "their head and its functions; with excretory functions; with genital functions"—in essence with their bodies (Glud & Blane, 1956, p. 30).

The emphasis on the head was reinforced by the use of the overhead mirror. Pugh and Tagiuri (1954) reported that those who used an overhead mirror while in the tank respirator viewed themselves as "heads", since the body was hidden by the tank. The mouth was seen as the most significant part of the head and one part of the body that was under the patient's control. It was the main source of communication and satisfaction.

Patients reported feeling different from others as a result of their experiences. Although most psychological imprints were associated with the "iron lung," the other mechanical breathing devices also became part of the new and often distorted self-images. For example, children who used a chest respirator (a protective plastic covering) often referred to themselves as "Space Men," revealing their sense of looking odd and different.

The sense of the body's integrity was also challenged by dependency on mechanical breathing devices. People usually think things happen to others. With the attack of polio, this sense of invulnerability was shattered.

The idea of being an "athlete", a "bread-winner", or a "house-wife" had been altered. Thoughts of being strong, pretty, or invincible lost their meaning. Many patients became depressed, as they began to feel that they could no longer live up to their dreams or aspirations.

Body image was affected, as well, if the patient needed to have a tracheotomy to help with breathing. Personality changes related to feelings of mutilation occurred, often leading to anxiety and depression, as people worried about their future.

Depersonalization.   Polio survivors have described having had feelings that they were outside of their bodies, looking at themselves, watching what was happening from above, feeling that it was not happening to them. This phenomenon is the psychological defense *depersonalization*, e.g., the sense that the body or parts of the body are not part of oneself. It is a way of psychologically distancing oneself from a traumatic event that threatens the body's integrity—an event that is associated with fears of suffering and annihilation.

The feelings of depersonalization or dissociation, which occurred particularly when in the iron lung, may reappear years later. Sometimes they recur when a survivor has to undergo surgery and is given an anesthetic, or when he or she needs mechanical assistance for breathing again. Even the thought of needing assisted ventilation for the post-polio symptoms could trigger feelings of depersonalization. Patients may fear they are going "crazy" when experiencing these sensations, and those treating them may unfortunately agree—not realizing that this is a residual of a psychological defense from years ago.

MENTAL STATUS CHANGES

As we have discussed, many patients suffered psychological disturbances, as a result of polio's attack on their respiratory system. Those not properly prepared for being placed in a tank respirator became overwhelmed or completely disorganized. Glud and Blane, writing at the time (1956), described this as a clouding of the senses. The clouding came from shallow breathing and carbon dioxide retention, which affected the higher centers of the brain and lead to periods of hyperactivity, vagueness, disorientation, and anxiety. Some patients had frightening dreams and hallucinations that they could not distinguish from reality.

Post-polio patients often express concern over their lapses of memory for much of their early treatment. Needless to say, given the high level of stress and disorientation, partial or complete amnesia is not uncommon. Unfortunately, in those years, there were not enough trained psychologists or other mental health professionals available to help patients deal with these disturbing experiences.

GUIDELINES FOR PHYSICIANS AND SIGNIFICANT OTHERS

Sometimes those with PPS begin to experience breathing problems. For those who had been ventilator-dependent in the past, the fear of having to be in that situation again can be overwhelming. For polio survivors, who are currently ventilator dependent, there is the fear of losing what respiratory function they now have and facing uncertain death.

Some cautions are in order for physicians and significant others:

1. Do not jump to conclusions when those with PPS seem to be "over-reacting". Be aware that they may be emotionally reliving feelings from the past, in addition to making adjustments in the present. Be supportive and try to be understanding; avoid minimizing what they are going through.

2. Do not assume because new improved ventilation devices are available that people will accept them readily. Memories from the past will set up resistances, at least initially.

3. Do not make the mistake of saying: "Well you've been on a ventilator before, so this will be nothing new for you." Do not assume that familiarity lessens anxiety; indeed, on the contrary, it often enhances it.

4. Do not jump to conclusions about peoples' noncompliance, argumentativeness, or other difficult behavior. Part of this behavior is fear; part is resistance to becoming dependent again, and a large part is a wish to avoid the medical world.

SELF-CONCEPT AND PERSONALITY

7

THE POLIO PERSONALITY: DOES IT EXIST?

People often ask if there is a "Polio Personality". My simple answer is: "Not that I've seen."

Those with polio come in all stripes, as they say. Some are ambitious, others more laid back, some have up-beat personalities, and some are depressed.

Polio affected people in different ways, physically, psychologically, and socially. Those who got polio came from different home environments. They went to different institutions for treatment and had different treatments. And they also had different educational and social opportunities and experiences. The list goes on and on, with each factor interacting with the others, shaping the person.

That said—the more complex answer recognizes that there is still some common ground that polio survivors share. Although there may not be a specific polio personality or a specific polio self-concept, the stories of others may sound familiar, and you may find yourself reacting in a similar way.

Let us look at one personality type that is common, though not universal.

THE DOER

Many polio survivors describe themselves as Doers. They are the ones who spend a lot of time taking care of others—family and friends. (At this point you may be smiling and shaking your head in recognition.)

The need to take care of others may come from guilt felt over the years, for having relied on others so much. "Doing" may be a defense that is intended to lessen the sense of guilt and help you feel accepted. In moderation "doing" can be a good thing, but when it takes on a life of its own and becomes "over-"doing", it can become a problem unto itself.

Maria, a self-reported Doer, says that even when she gets tired, she is not able to stop herself:

"I just keep on "doing", until I'm fatigued—and then I become resentful."

"I do too much for people and come on too strong.

"I try to fix others. If I can fix others, I don't have to focus on myself."

HELPING THE DOER NOT TO OVER-DO

Take a piece of paper and write down the WHYS and WHATS:

1. Why do you feel you have to keep going?
2. What are you afraid of?
3. What do you think others will think of you if you don't keep going and "doing" more?
4. Why do you care?

5. What would happen if you weren't so helpful anymore, if you just stopped?

6. What may you be avoiding in looking at yourself?

THE TYPE A PERSONALITY AND PPS: FACT OR WHAT?

Let us not confuse the Doer with the Type A personality. Do polio survivors have Type A personalities? Some seem to think so, since many of those who survived polio are real strivers and doers so to speak. But before we reach any conclusions we need to understand what is meant by Type A.

Type A and Type B Personalities

People typically think of those with Type A personalities, as very active, ambitious, hardworking, and successful. But this is not the whole story.

The Type A personality is characterized by

- aggressiveness,
- competitiveness, and
- impatience.

It has been described as the "hurry sickness." Those so classified are easily moved to

- anger

and show frequent displays of

- irritation, and
- hostility,

particularly when things are not moving fast enough nor going, as they would like.

This is in contrast to the Type B personality, which is more relaxed and more accepting of life and of others.

RESEARCH FINDINGS

Early studies of Type A personality looked at the relationship of this personality syndrome to heart attacks. The implication of the findings was that a person's Type A personality caused the heart attacks. That is still the idea in the popular press, even though more recent research is showing the issue to be much more complex.

Results are mixed and seem to depend upon the different questionnaires and interview techniques used to assess Type A traits. It does appear, however, that certain traits, such as *anger, hostility, cynicism, and suspiciousness* affect a person's tendency to succumb to some illnesses.

The polio literature often refers to those with post-polio syndrome (PPS) as having Type A personalities. If we accept this, are we then saying that those who had polio are typically hostile and angry, cynical and suspicious? I think not. Some may be, but is this the rule? Having a little bit or some of the traits does not mean one is Type A.

Amongst those who had the gumption to try psychotherapy with me, some survivors did exhibit Type A traits. But I cannot say that this was in greater proportion than in the general population. And there were certainly those with more "laid back" attitudes and behaviors, typical of the Type B personality.

More research needs to be done before one can make statements with confidence about the relationship between personality and PPS. In so doing, we must be careful that our surveys are not biased.

Those who participate in research studies are quite possibly a select group. Because of their character traits, survivors with Type A traits are the ones most likely to turn up at support groups or to seek help from clinics and physicians. They are more assertive, for example, than those who stay home and do not seek help for their problems. They are also more likely to answer questionnaires in greater numbers than their Type B counterparts, who are, thus, not well represented in our data.

Why is This Important?

One reason is the common belief that over-doing it physically may have contributed to post-polio symptoms. After all, the treatment early on was to exercise, exercise, exercise, and exercise. And throughout life for many there was the continued pressure to be like others, to succeed, if not excel, in the mainstream. Do; do more; do more and more.

Still some hearing about the possible association between Type A and polio may worry: Did I cause my post-polio symptoms? Did all that exercise and activity throughout my life lead to PPS?

A BAD RAP

The Type A personality has been given a bad rap. It is not something to be ashamed of, nor is it necessarily something to be changed. In some cases, it may be a very good type of personality to have, as long as certain traits, such as hostility and anger, are kept under control.

Persons with Type A are often very successful in their lives, and in terms of heart attacks do much better than their counterpart Type B's when it comes to surviving a second heart attack. Some think it is the very Type A traits that enable people to take better care of their health following the first attack. Thus, it may be a good thing that some survivors of polio have the assertiveness and energy so common to the Type A; this may be what makes them seek better medical care and be active in keeping the medical profession on its toes.

PPS AND TYPE A

So what does this mean in terms of the person who has had polio? Did the earlier efforts in treatment cause people to become Type A's? Certainly there was pressure to exercise and to be reintegrated into society at large. Yet in my clinical experience I cannot say that all those who had polio or have PPS fit the classic Type A description. Indeed, many lead successful busy lives, but others were not so fortunate. Those who were successful may have been ambitious, but not necessarily hostile or angry.

Having polio or developing new symptoms can make one angry at times. Being frustrated by physicians who do not understand can bring out hostile feelings, even in the most eventempered. But these feelings or behaviors alone do not make a Type A. In fact it may be the keeping in of hostile feelings that compromises one's health. The issue is very complex, as we've said before.

Labeling may be useful in research when one is grouping large numbers of people for studies. But labeling individuals can be misleading, inaccurate and possibly harmful. If people who had polio—or for that matter, cancer, MS, or other diseases—are made to feel that their personalities are the cause of their physical problems, that is another burden put upon them.

By overusing the term Type A, we obscure what the experience and behavior of those with PPS is really about—interfering with our deeper understanding of the late effects of polio.

8

SELF-CONCEPT AND PPS

As we have discussed, there is no particular "polio personality". And in the same vein, survivors have no characteristic polio self-concept. However, those who had polio find they share some similar experiences that still affect their sense of self.

As a polio survivor, your self-concept was formed in part by your earlier experiences with polio, and in recent years your self-esteem may have taken a battering from the new symptoms and problems that emerge with post-polio syndrome (PPS).

—How you feel physically, and what you can do or not do, play an important role in how you see yourself.

—Changes in your body and in your appearance affect your body image and how you feel about who you are.

You can feel good about yourself, or you can feel down on yourself. Your self-concept can be a motivator for change, or it can be what holds you back and makes you hide from others.

CHANGES IN THE SENSE OF SELF: SEX DIFFERENCES

Women and men differ in their reactions to their PPS symptoms. This gender difference is not uncommon in medicine and psychology. Society has conditioned women and men to see themselves in certain ways; thus, they have different ways of experiencing illness and of expressing their needs.

In a small study that I conducted on the effects of age and PPS, survivors reported that their sense of self had changed since they started getting post-polio symptoms.

Although both sexes reported a change in sense of self, they used different words to express their experiences.

Over all men and women saw themselves as being *less energetic*.

However, men described themselves *as very impatient* and *more irritable*.

Women, on the other hand, saw themselves as *hard working*, but *less active* and *more depressed*.

For men, underlying the change in the sense of self is an increasing *lack of self-confidence*. This is related to the many *physical losses* that take place with PPS, and the recognition that you are not able to do things as before.

Men suffer a lessening of self-esteem and a lack of identity, when they find themselves no longer able to work. One man reported feeling *"less manly"*, as he was unable to support his family as in the past and was not as physically strong and active as before.

In many cases sexuality and sexual prowess are diminished, although this is an area that is not easily talked about. Over time PPS requires a series of adjustments coupled with an increasing dependency on others. New ailments and a fear of what the future holds add an element of anxiety to the mix.

The women's reports were of a different sort. A common complaint was feeling *less attractive* than before, reflecting the societal pressure on women to be pretty. One woman commented on *how difficult it is to feel successful.* Another was frustrated with not being able to dress herself or take care of basic necessities. Another woman got angry with herself for not being as active as she used to be, an internalization of the anger—which is not uncommon for women in general.

And another woman summed it up this way:

> *"Sometimes I feel a sense of worthlessness and sadness that goes all the way to my soul. I try to enjoy each day fully. Some days are OK, and some days are very hard."*

POSITIVE THINKING

Despite the difficulties, many, if not most, survivors feel generally good about themselves and their lives. That doesn't mean that they feel as energetic or as attractive as in their youth. At times hurtful things do happen or are said. But having a positive image of oneself helps you to weather the rough spots.

But when you are in the doldrums you may wonder: What do I have to feel good about?

Many survivors feel good about themselves for helping others. Even though we may see the DOER as potentially someone who overdoes, there is a certain reward that comes from helping others. There is also a sense of competence that comes from the practice of taking charge and knowing that you can handle things.

Those who are active in polio support groups find the experience rewarding. Oh, there are the frustrating times that come when dealing with other people. But on the whole, the mission of the support group—helping other survivors cope and educating doctors and the public—can give you a sense of purpose in life and a sense of accomplishment.

Having raised a family or been an active member of a family (even if you didn't have your own children) can enhance your sense of self. The rewards that come from seeing the results of your efforts take shape over time and add to your positive self-concept.

Some people find fulfillment in their jobs, depending upon what they do and the responsibilities that they have. In some cases, people with polio have developed and worked in their own businesses. Although on the day-to-day level such work can be difficult at times, overall seeing what you have developed and achieved can make you feel quite proud.

Retirement, however, with extra time on your hands, can present problems:

> What to do with your time;
> Questioning who you are;
> What you have done with your life;
> What to do with the rest of your life.

This is true for retirees in general, not just those with PPS. Finding a way to stay active and feel competent may require a new identity, new interests, leading to new achievements.

Some achieve a renewed sense of self by furthering their education, be it in a formal setting or reading and studying on their own. Hobbies and sports are other venues that help you feel positive about life. Spending time with family has it rewards.

Many polio survivors take great pride in knowing that they have overcome many obstacles in their lives; some feel overwhelmed by all the challenges that they have had to face and still must face. But they tell themselves that having succeeded in life thus far, they know they will face the challenges that await them. They use their positive sense of self to help them carry on.

OTHER-DIRECTED VS INNER-DIRECTED

As a polio survivor, your self-concept was formed in part by your earlier experiences with polio. Your self-concept can be a motivator for change, or it can be what holds you back and makes you hide from others. You can feel good about yourself, or you can feel down on yourself.

Walter, a polio survivor, remembers feeling "grateful" when people wanted to be with him:

"I was so happy when someone invited me to play."

He expected to be overlooked, rejected, patronized, and just plain ignored. As a result, Walter now feels that he has become someone who always wants to please, which means that he often doesn't evaluate people very well.

Thus, begins a vicious cycle that leaves him open to those who may not be sensitive or caring, people who take advantage of his need to please. Since he has trouble standing up for himself, Walter sets himself up for the very things he fears: rejection, isolation, and being used.

As a result Walter always feels bad about himself. He feels as if he's not doing enough or is not good enough.

"I've acted grateful and appreciative my whole life. And I know now that I did it out of fear.

Sometimes I act independent just to keep others away."

INTERNALIZING THE REACTIONS OF OTHERS

Like Walter, much of your self-concept may be "other-directed," a term coined in 1961 by the sociologist, David Riesman, in his classic book, "The Lonely Crowd". By this he means:

> How we see ourselves in relation to how we think others perceive us.

Notice the word "think" in that definition, as it is critical. We may project onto others thoughts they don't even have, thoughts that come from our own concerns and worries. Yet the perceived reactions of others, both positive and negative, help shape our self-concept throughout our lives.

If you are very "other-directed," you read peoples' reactions as you would a mirror; checking on how you look, what is good, what is bad; how you've changed. You become hyper-vigilant, checking every nuance and reading things into everything others say or do. You may have internalized voices from the past criticizing you, teasing you, perhaps telling you that you are bad.

"The Look of Pity"

Bernice is other-directed. Her life is focused on what the other person is thinking. One of the things she fears most is "the look of pity". She asks herself:

> *"What about me makes them glance away or adopt that strange look?"*

Maybe someone is thinking "that poor soul"—a thought that, if you feel like Bernice, may bother you a lot. You don't want to be pitied. But some days you may pity yourself, wondering, "Why me?"

Seeing what you interpret as pity in someone else's face triggers the pity you have buried somewhere inside of you. The rage you feel is not only with what you feel is their insensitivity, but it is an expression of your own, at times fragile, self-concept—a rage against yourself and your situation.

Notice that Bernice asks what is it "about me." Maybe it isn't all about her. She may not be the issue, only the catalyst. Perhaps she should have phrased it this way: *"What is it that makes people stare?"*

Yes, it is true that many people do stare at people who have a disability, but they may have their own issues or thoughts that you are not aware of.

Maybe they do feel sorry for you. But maybe they are just curious, possibly admiring how you get around. Perhaps they are interested in seeing how you manage, in case they find themselves in the same situation one day; they would know what to do.

Although it can be tiring and annoying to notice people's unease, your inner sense of self needs to come alive and answer that question with a positive response.

> *"It's not about me, it's about them.*
> *I will not let my negative thoughts deter me."*

What you say to yourself, and how you feel about yourself define how you will react…and sometimes how others will react to you.

Accepting Praise: The Conflict

Bonnie has trouble accepting praise. She feels that people "over-praise" you when you have a disability. This was especially true when she was a child but still goes on now, particularly at work.

> *"Because you are disabled, they tell you that whatever you do is good. They have different standards for disabled people.*
>
> *This makes it hard to judge yourself or others. You have no sense of other people's sincerity and a distorted sense of who you really are."*

Bonnie goes on to explain:

> *"Sometimes people make me feel that I have to be heroic. I guess I'm supposed to be like Wonder Woman.*
>
> *And then they say to themselves: 'Thank you for not making us feel bad.' It's like a no-win situation."*

DEVELOPING A POSITIVE INNER VOICE

However, some people are more "inner-directed" than "other-directed." Such people are more likely to heed their own internal voice, which has its own core of values. They are less likely to be influenced by others, having what is often called a strong ego.

Most people, however, are a little of each.

Where does this inner direction come from? In many cases, the fortunate people have had others who encouraged them from a young age and rewarded them with genuine compliments and encouragement. They internalized what they heard and made it theirs.

In later years as adults, they were able to draw upon these positive voices to stay focused on their strengths and the rewarding aspects of their lives.

Even survivors who have had few rewarding experiences in the past can be driven by a strong inner sense of self. They learn to listen to positive voices from within and without, choosing carefully whose words to believe and whose to discard.

You need to:

- Focus on the positive steps that you have taken in life, no matter how small or seemingly insignificant.

- Give yourself permission to recognize your accomplishments.

- Learn to see the glass as half full, not have empty, as the saying goes.

This is not to turn you into a Pollyanna-type individual. In being inner-directed you do recognize the challenges of life, but you use this self-talk to encourage yourself to try, to go on, and not to be bogged down by self criticism.

SOCIAL ENCOUNTERS

9

HELP: LEARNING TO GIVE AND TO RECEIVE

GETTING THE HELP YOU NEED: THE CONFLICTS

You may find that your stamina and strength aren't what they used to be. This means that you now need to ask others for help with tasks that you used to do easily, like reaching, lifting, bending, or carrying.

Figuring out
—when to ask,
—whom to ask, and
—how to ask
can be trying

ASKING FOR HELP: THE FRUSTRATIONS

"I hate having to wait on others' good will and timing, especially when I need something done that I used to be able to do myself."

This complaint is usually directed at a spouse or significant other, who is busy doing something else, such as, reading an article in the newspaper or looking for something on the Internet.

The wait, even when just a few minutes, can be very frustrating. What you are asking for wouldn't take much time, you tell yourself. And you need it right now. For your spouse, however, it means interrupting a train of thought or losing something that he or she has been working on for some time.

However, having to ask over and over can test your patience. Asking and waiting serve to highlight the increasing loss of function that worries you, and the loss of independence that depresses and frightens you. The fright can turn into rage directed at yourself and at the other person and even lead you to question if anyone really cares or comprehends what you are going through.

Those who do not have a disability do not understand what you go through every day. They may minimize your feelings, perhaps telling you that you are too impatient, or they may compliment you on how strong you are and how brave. The dismissive comments, as well as the well-intentioned compliments, set up conflicting feelings inside you.

GUIDELINES: WHEN AND HOW TO ASK

Learning **how** to ask for help and **when** to ask for help are both important, if you are to control stress in your life and get your needs met.

If you need help, ask. Take a chance. If you are refused, examine the situation to see what you could do differently the next time:

- Put yourself in the other person's shoes.
- Think about how you might react if the situation were reversed.

- Compliment rather than criticize.

If the help you want doesn't come right away, stop your negative thoughts:

- Set your priorities. Be willing to wait, if possible.
- Try to think of other ways to view the situation.

    Sometimes the other person is just plain tired, or simply didn't hear you. Particularly now that we are all aging, a person's hearing may not be what it once was. So a nod of the head does not necessarily mean that the person really heard you or understood all that you said.

    But admittedly, there are those who are just plain ornery and only do things when they feel like it!

THE KINDNESS OF STRANGERS

Knowing how to get help *when you need it* is very tricky. The memorable quote from the Tennessee Williams' play, *Streetcar Named Desire,* has Blanche DuBois saying—in this case proudly and longingly: "I always rely on the kindness of strangers."

However, for most polio survivors, it is not that easy to ask for help. Some see Blanche DuBois' reliance on others, particularly strangers, as pathetic. To others dependency comes to mind and overwhelms them with fear. But it does not need to be so. Relying on others is sometimes a necessary part of life.

Vanessa, a quite independent polio survivor, drives her adapted van all over the city where she lives. However, she still needs help putting her wheelchair back into her van.

Her strategy is to stand by the parked vehicle, scrutinizing everyone who goes by, looking for a strong healthy person (usually a youngish male). Then she zeros in on him making her request.

Vanessa says she makes a game out of this, and has never been turned down, as she appeals to "their young male egos".

DEALING WITH OFFERS OF HELP

A typical complaint is that people, particularly strangers, offer help when help isn't wanted. Of course, those doing the offering can be in a quandary. They may want to be helpful, but are not sure what to do. Some just give up and don't bother, thus coming off as uncaring.

Those who do offer may feel rebuffed if their offer of help is rejected, especially if the rejection is done in a brusque way. What they don't realize is that you may have spent a good part of your outing just trying to be on your own, while others are trying to be in your life helping you.

Some strangers just take the risk and offer anyway, leaving you with another person to whom you either say, "Yes, thank you", or "No, thank you"—perhaps for the umpteenth time. Yes, it does get to you sometimes.

Accepting help from others is a complicated matter. It is not just related to the awkward social interactions with strangers mentioned above. Carol describes well the conflicts she and many others have in accepting help. On one hand she says:

"What is lacking in my life is someone extending a hand to me. But when people do try to help, I am uncomfortable; I'm afraid it is not meant, not sincere.

"I send out the message: 'Don't help me; I don't need your help'.

"I can't ask for help. I see needing help as a sign of weakness.

"I feel like I've failed as a person, if I can't do things on my own. Needing help makes me feel worthless.

"If I need help, people won't love me. I'll be discarded. They'll keep me around as a friend, but with disdain."

GUIDELINES: GRACIOUS MANAGING OF OFFERS OF HELP

So what to do when people offer to help?

- If you need the help that is offered, then accept it without self-incriminations. Don't make your life harder than it is, and don't go on and on apologizing for being a burden.

- Say thank-you…but don't overdo it by saying "Thank-you" over and over for every little thing.

- Remember to reward the person who offers to help you with a smile and some kindnesses of your own. One gets further with positive reinforcement than with negative. So even if you don't need help right now, you might later, so you don't want to turn the helpers off completely.

- If you really don't want any help and can manage on your own, just say so, and add, "Thanks for asking." That way the other person will not be embarrassed or put off, and may at another time extend a hand to someone else who could actually use some help.

10

THE NEED FOR BOUNDARIES

The following stories appeared on an Internet chat forum and raise some interesting questions.

"I was in a flea market the other day in my wheelchair where I noticed a man about my age who had the same polio residual as I before the PPS [post-polio syndrome] left my leg limp. So I asked him—a complete stranger, how nervy of me—if he was having symptoms of PPS.

"Well he looked at me like I had hexed him, like I put a curse on him. But he did answer that he was experiencing extreme fatigue. So I told him about the PPS group, the research, etc. All he could say was, 'Did you see a psychiatrist?'

"I totally understand his state of denial and maybe the dawning of an awareness. So I just cautioned him to rest, save his strength, and plan for the worst and the best will happen. We just parted on that note. He was definitely frightened of the unknown."

Another writer on the same chat forum described an angry encounter with another man who resisted "advice":

"I do not want to know anymore, thank you. My wife had enough of polio when she was young, and she wants nothing to do with anyone and their wacky notions. And no, we don't want to go on any mailing list."

This raises the questions:

How do we approach the subject of PPS without upsetting anyone?

How do we know when we have invaded another's personal space and our help is not wanted?

How do we stop others from invading our personal space?

ON SHARING INFORMATION

In both of these incidents it may be that the advice-givers were not sensitive to the needs of others. They were like proselytizers who felt they had the Word, the answers. But people do not always appreciate others' enthusiasm, even when the advice-giver may have something to say. The first man's asking if the advice-giver had seen a psychiatrist, leads me to suspect that the "helper" was going on and on, without any sensitivity to the other's willingness to participate. Your wishing to share information may be a noble intention, but what you have to say is not in itself "helpful", if the other person is not ready or willing to listen.

What if you really feel that you have information that the other may benefit from? You need to go slow to see how each step you take is accepted. You need to be aware of the others' boundaries and recognize resistance as a sign to back off.

You also need to be aware of your own motives: Perhaps it is you who is frightened, and by bonding with others it makes you feel better. Perhaps being knowledgeable makes you feel important, or more in control of your own PPS.

Maybe you just genuinely want to help others and genuinely feel that you know the way. However, if your good intentions begin to penetrate others' personal boundaries, you will make them uncomfortable. Feeling violated, they may lash out at you in anger. As with the advice-givers in the chat sites above, you may say that the resistant other is in denial, but it may be you, the advice-giver, who has the unmet needs.

What About Denial?

The resistance that comes between you and the person you are trying to engage may indeed be a function of denial. And if so, is that bad? In our discussion in the chapter on Psychological Defenses we take a close look at the role of denial as a coping mechanism, in both its healthy and unhealthy forms.

Denial as a defense gives people time and distance to help them cope with stressful situations. When not overdone, it is not always bad.

So as a layperson, be careful when labeling people with psychological terms. Sometimes defenses are helping others cope with difficult situations. In other cases, it may not be denial; it may be them just keeping you out, not wanting to discuss their private lives with you.

PERSONAL BOUNDARIES

In life we need boundaries to function: Boundaries between parents and children, between the sexes, between strangers, between friends, between family members, and yes, even between spouses. People have different needs in terms of their life spaces and how comfortable they are in letting others be close to them.

In this age of sharing and bearing all on TV talk shows, we may have lost some of the sense of personal boundaries. It is OK, even necessary, to set limits around your personal space. But in the same vein it is important not only to know your own boundaries but also to be respectful of those of others.

Many people are not happy talking about their personal problems, including medical and physical disabilities. And to talk about them to strangers or mere acquaintances can be experienced as an unwanted intrusion into their personal lives, their privacy. Such talk may make them anxious or embarrassed, or they may just be very private and keep things to themselves and maybe a small circle of others.

The right to privacy still exists in this age of openness. Put yourself in others' shoes. Remember the times that you thought others were staring at you? When someone asked you: "What happened to you?" When you felt self-conscious or were tired of thinking about your problems. Sometimes you just don't want to focus on PPS. It is a nice day. You just want to be in it; you want to enjoy it. No serious talk.

SETTING LIMITS

Friends and acquaintances can ask intrusive questions, some people can really be quite persistent. You question their motives and sincerity. You wonder if they are judging you. You don't want to be the center of attention. You wonder, "Why are they being so nosey?"

What if the person asking questions is a total stranger, and what if he or she offers advice? How do you know if you should take it?

On the other hand, it is sometimes easier to talk to a stranger. Have you not had long conversations with strangers on a bus or train, where you have felt free to open up? Maybe it's because you know inside that you will never see that person again. You don't have to worry about what you say. You get the release from talking about your feelings and the complications in your life, and you may even gain some insight. Yet you still maintain some control over when you want to talk about these things again. The person you are talking to won't be there tomorrow to remind you of what you said today.

It should be your choice when to enter into personal conversations. Yet how do you handle invasive questions? You've been told not to lie, but sometimes a "white lie" is all that you can muster to get out of an awkward spot. To tell all, to tell a bit, or to ignore the question: Which way to go?

GUIDELINES: WARDING OFF INTRUSIVE OTHERS

Have a few prepared sentences, such as:

"Thank-you for your interest, but I'd rather not talk about that now."

Whatever your prepared responses are, practice them in your head periodically, so when someone gets close to your personal limits, you can respond calmly and politely—not with an irritated edge to your voice. If they persist, as some do, repeat your phrase again till they get the message. If they think you are in denial, so be it. You cannot control others' thinking.

GUIDELINES:
MANAGING YOUR HELPFUL INSTINCTS

When you hit resistance, back off. It is not up to you to diagnose someone's behavior or feelings or to solve another person's psychological problems. Leave that to the professionals.

If you have the urge to help others with PPS, you can reach out to them through G.I.N.I. and through your local support group. Donate your time and money, if you can. Most support groups have lots of members who like to offer advice. But what they need are reliable people to help them with the administrative detail work and the organizational work. It may not feel directly rewarding, but it is necessary. Volunteer, even if you have to do it from home.

11

CHANGING ROLES: SURVIVORS' PERSPECTIVES

AGING AND PPS

Haven't you noticed that as people age those little idiosyncrasies that you were able to ignore have now become more rigid and more pronounced—and more irritating? Maybe even your idiosyncrasies are showing. Have you noticed that you are becoming more like your mother or your father—possibly showing those traits and behaviors that you thought were funny or annoying?

And with age haven't you noticed your strength changing, particularly if you are not keeping yourself fit? But keeping fit is harder to do if you have mobility or breathing problems related to post-polio syndrome (PPS). And of course your eyesight and hearing may not what they used to be, not to mention your memory. Remember your mind needs exercise too.

So as we grow older, we change and our roles naturally change. Add PPS to the mix, and you will see that *PPS complicates all the ordinary issues of life.*

Thus, with these unwelcome changes:

- Some must learn to do more
- Some must learn to do less,

     and

- Some won't want to do either.

The effects of aging cannot be separated from PPS, as they are intertwined, affecting all aspects of your psychological and social being. So with age the questions come: How will I take care of myself? Who will help me? How do I deal with all these challenges that are being thrust into my life?

NEW EXPECTATIONS AND FRUSTRATIONS

As PPS symptoms progress, survivors' roles within the family begin to change. Needless to say, this causes stress for all concerned.

The first symptoms of PPS come on gradually, but they are often attributed to other things. Survivors find that they no longer have the stamina or strength to do what they once did; they may need to cut down on their activities or ask for help from others—*God forbid.* I say the last somewhat in jest, as learning to ask for help is one of the most troubling issues for many polio survivors.

The recognition that your body is not what it once was can be quite unsettling. You feel betrayed by your body. Since in the past you were told to try, try, and continue trying, you may expect that, if you just keep pushing, you'll be able to do all the things that you used to do. But alas, as PPS progresses, this may not be possible. Bit-by-bit you may have to modify your habits and rearrange your responsibilities, turning some over to others.

WORK AND FINANCES

You may have to cut back on your activities. If you have been working, the time for change may come sooner than you like. You may be faced with having to have your work modified to meet your needs. Often this accommodation can be made with not much difficulty. However, in some situations it may be quite complicated to work out—and in doing so you may draw attention to yourself—something you really would rather avoid.

As your weakness progresses and other symptoms begin to appear, you may have to find other ways to get to work, or to work less, or to work from home. Your income may be affected by these changes, putting more stress on you and your family. How to find supplementary income then becomes another challenge. Financial pressures can mount, even for those who are relatively financially well off.

Within the family, the pattern gets played out again. If you were contributing to your family's support you may not be able to do so anymore, at least not as much as before. Another family member may have to go to work now—willingly or perhaps not so willingly. Or the converse, an employed spouse may need to stay home to take care of the person who has PPS. Someone may need to be hired for housekeeping, adding to the financial pressures. New concerns mount: How to get financial help, SSI, or assistive devices? How to modify the home? All this takes research and time.

You may tell yourself that you will deal with these issues, if or when the need arises. Sometimes, however, the changes sneak up on you, and you have no time to really plan. Or perhaps you have just been ignoring them, hoping that somehow you could continue as you've been. But then you are faced with the realities of what you can and can no longer do.

NEW LIFESTYLES IN RETIREMENT

Today many people with PPS are retired. They may have retired from a job because they reached retirement age, or gone out on disability. Just being at home without structure can cause tension between people who live together. They have to learn to have their own interests and to know when to share these interests with others. But the things you used to dream about doing, when you wouldn't have to work anymore, may not now be possible. For one, you may not be able to do them without assistance from others. And asking for help is not what you had in mind.

Chores and responsibilities at home begin to be divided differently. Maybe you used to do the yard work, but now have to give more and more of those chores to others. No raking leaves, weeding, carrying heavy objects. If you did most of the housekeeping, someone else may have to take over those duties. Such change does not come easily.

ROLE CHANGES AND THE FAMILY

Family members may not recognize that you can no longer do what you used to do. They may urge you to keep trying, by saying "You can do it." Perhaps they believe that by encouraging you they are helping you not to give up. Sometimes this is good, but sometimes this comes from a misunderstanding of what you are going through, what you can do, or what you really should be doing.

For example, other people may have gotten use to your doing all the housework and become resentful that they are now being asked to chip in. They may never have liked doing things around the house, and see this responsibility as an added burden. Such a situation can cause tension at home, as things don't get done.

If you were the primary housekeeper, you may have had a way that you used to like to have things done. You may still put in your two-cents, but only to the annoyance of others, be they your spouse or children, who are taking over new chores.

Sometimes people, who don't like doing certain tasks, are able to swallow their resentment when they realize that they are being of help to someone else or to the common good. This feeling comes easily to some, but can take some time to develop for others.

Fun things may have changed too. Perhaps you used to take walks with family members, and now can't. Or maybe bicycling together was a big part of your life, and you can no longer do that. Finding other common areas takes effort. And as the PPS progresses, over time you may have to change again to find more outlets for creativity and relaxing, and having fun as a family.

A person plays many different roles in the family and outside of the family. Letting go of the old roles and working out the details of the new ones can cause a lot of stress, both physically and emotionally. Changes in ideas and patterns that have been established over a lifetime do not come without some psychological struggle.

PERSONAL RELATIONSHIPS

12

CHILDREN

YOUR CHILDREN AND YOUR PPS

Children can be a mixed blessing, particularly where post-polio syndrome (PPS) is involved. In some families they are supportive and understanding; in others there is anger and a sense of frustration on both sides.

In many cases the way children react to their parents depends upon their age. Young children are quite conformist, despite all their antics. They want their parents to be like their friends' parents. They want their parents to blend in and not to draw attention. The fear of humiliation is great. In young people being different means being teased, not fitting in and being rejected. Those who had polio when young can well identify with these concerns.

Now that those with PPS are older, their children have moved into adulthood. But the children may bring with them their concerns from the past. The problems of acceptance may still continue but express themselves in different ways.

Children of any age may have difficulty facing the fearful reality of a parent's having a debilitating condition. This goes for the older children as well. Not only is a parent's vulnerability frightening to contemplate, it also brings to consciousness one's own sense of vulnerability and mortality.

But on a more practical level the adult children also have many other responsibilities: the running of their own home, raising their own children and grandchildren, and their work. Faced with a parent's increased weakness due to PPS, they begin to feel the stress of taking on more responsibility. Thus, the defense of denial may set in. They may not want to know or may be afraid to know.

For example, sometimes your children may act as if they don't hear you, when you say you are tired. After all you don't look much different than before. They try to encourage you to keep doing what you used to do.

After all, this is the generation that jogs all the time and works out at 5:30 in the morning. More is not enough for them. And so what looks like "not listening", may just be their extending to you their own coping behaviors. Or are they just modeling what they've learned from watching you over the years, which was what you learned during your first treatments for polio? Do more, do more. Push, push.

One common complaint is that children *do not offer to help unless asked, and then do so reluctantly.* As we know, many with PPS do not like to ask for help, so when they do ask, it means they have muscled up a lot of courage. The guilt they feel increases, when they must ask over and over. This guilt gradually turns to anger, when the requests are met with resistance. The anger is often not expressed, and instead is turned inward, leading to an increase in depression and physical problems related to stress.

Ada, a single parent, cried as she told me that her son, when in high school, was embarrassed to be seen with her. She had "a limp" and had difficulty walking as fast as others. Later when he was applying to colleges, he did not want her to go with him to Visiting Day at the campuses.

He told his mother that he would be embarrassed because she would not be able to keep up with the other parents on their tour of the school. Also, she would not be able to climb stairs and would have to ask for special considerations. In other words, they would be different and call attention to themselves. Ada cried when she told me this story, even though it had happened many years before.

In her son's mind the attention would be negative. But that is not necessarily the case. Seeing a caring son with a disabled mother may have been a feather in his cap. And seeing a disabled mother going about doing all the things a mother is expected to do would be a feather in both their caps and possibility an enlightening experience for the college administrators and the others applying to the school.

Needless to say not all children are this outspoken or cruel to their parents. However, many teenagers and those older feel some of what this young man expressed. How they handle their feelings depends in large part upon how they were brought up. In this particular case, there were difficulties with the father over the years that played into the son's taking his anger out on his mother. Ada came to understand this, which helped to lessen the pain that she felt, but she could not forget what he said.

As illustrated here, some of these hurtful behaviors may be "normal" or understandable on the part of children of certain ages, but they can have far reaching consequences. Over time parents struggling with the late effects of polio may need to turn to their children for support—and the early tensions may make these role changes less easy.

Children like all of us come with different personalities, so it is not possible to say, "Just do this and it will all work out." Although you may not always be successful all the time, you have to try to communicate with them about your needs and the changing conditions, at the same time recognizing that they have their fears and their own stresses.

You can share information about PPS with your children. Some will read it and others not. Some will believe it, and others will not.

In asking them to be understanding of your changing condition and the changing roles in the family, it is also important for you to hear them—to hear about the demands on them and what your new needs mean to them. These are real concerns for your children no matter how you perceive the situation. It is important that their concerns be taken into account when looking for new solutions. Sometimes you may realize that you need to look beyond the family to get your needs met.

> Is there someone else who can drive you, someone else who can shop for you or take you to the doctor?
>
> Can you get the groceries delivered?
>
> Can you find someone to clean the house once in a while?
>
> Do you have access to a van to take you to your medical visits?

Your needs are real for you, but you must let your children see that you appreciate their needs too. Unlike in other cultures parents and children in the U.S. do not always live with each other or near each other. And when they do, they may still set personal boundaries in terms of their interactions. Sometimes this is a result of how things were in the past, like old hurts resurfacing, or feeling they did not get enough attention from you. Or as we've said, they most likely have many responsibilities or are having problems accepting what you are going through.

If you are fortunate and have a child or children who can be there for you, then remember to thank them—though not overly so, or you will make them uncomfortable. If the adult child cannot be around all the time for you, try not to lay guilt trips on them by telling them how lonely or needy you are. If you are lonely or needy, however, discuss this with them but do not expect them to be the sole solution. Let them help you find new social outlets or ways to take care of your daily activities.

GRANDCHILDREN: ANOTHER GENERATION

Many polio survivors are now of the age where they also have grandchildren or great grandchildren. These young folks grew up at a different time and in a different family constellation than their parents. They most likely accept the grandparents who have PPS as just who they are. There is not the same identification as between parent and child.

Yet the grandchildren too may not fully understand what you are going through with PPS. But they are less likely to have as intense conflicts as their parents have in regards to you.

These young folds can provide healthy distractions for the woes of aging and PPS. Depending upon their ages and how close they live, they may be able to provide some of the help that you need, which would also be a way of teaching them responsibility and empathy.

With both children and grandchildren, be careful not to ask them to spend more time with you than they obviously are interested in doing. Be glad that you have someone who is there for you as much as he or she can be. Otherwise they can become resentful and withdraw, which is the exact opposite of what you want.

13

PARENTS: THEN AND NOW

"We never talked about what happened," Alice complained to me. *"Sometimes I want to know and sometimes I'm not sure."*

Now that you are an adult and the symptoms of post-polio syndrome (PPS) are causing you to reflect on your early years, you find yourself having many questions about those days. This is particularly true if you were an infant or a young child when you had polio, and remember little or nothing of the experience.

If your parents are no longer alive—which is true for most polio survivors today—there may be no one to help you find the answers. You may feel cheated that they didn't tell you more. You may blame yourself for not asking more questions when you had the chance. But some subjects are not easy to bring up.

When they were alive, your parents may not have wanted to talk about that time, telling you they didn't remember, or that you shouldn't torment yourself thinking about things that are in the past.

If your parents did not want to talk to you now about what happened in those early years, it may be that they buried those painful memories and were afraid to bring them up later. They did not know if they would be able to talk about these stressful times without falling apart emotionally. Or perhaps they felt that you would blame them for not taking better care of you—feelings of guilt that they may have harbored, rightly or wrongly, over the years.

You may become angry, thinking that they were holding out on you, that they knew things that they didn't want to tell you. In the case of polio there was much that was not talked about. Was it out of shame? Guilt? Secrets were kept for fear that the child or the family would be ostracized, if others knew that there was polio in the family.

The belief was that one should just move on.

MEMORIES

If you were an infant when you had polio, you have no clear conscious memories of the events. There may be feelings that you can't seem to grasp—a low underlying anxiety, depression or fear. You really aren't sure what happened to you.

If you were older at the time polio struck, like so many survivors, you will have some memories from the past, though they may be fragmented. Since at the time you weren't told much about what was happening, you have been left with your own interpretation of what was going on.

Over the years you may have heard others talking about those early years, and by now you may not be sure what you really remember and what you think you remember. As you heard stories being told and retold, you developed mental images of the events described. Over time you can begin to believe that that mental images are things that you really experienced and really remember. But that is not always the case.

THE PAST:
PARENTS' REACTIONS AND EXPERIENCES

Put yourself back in time. Think about what it must have been like in the 1950's. It was not a time of talking about feelings, confronting physicians or demanding your rights in a hospital setting. Polio was being heralded in the press in much the same way that AIDS dominated the headlines in the late 20th century and beyond. Fear of contagion pervaded the general population.

Now that you can see this through adult eyes, ask yourself: What were your parents going through all this time? What were they feeling? What were their experiences?

Parental Reactions to Polio

Following the diagnosis of polio, parents reacted with acute anxiety and fear, which could turn into denial and disbelief. This reaction was particularly so, if at first the child did not appear to be very sick, as was the case with many who got polio. Guilt, shame, and sadness commonly followed, depending upon the circumstances.

Search for a Cause

"This can't be polio," would turn into the anguished question: *"How could my child get polio?"*

A search for the cause of the illness aroused all sorts of fantasies and explanations. Parents scrutinized every aspect of their child's life for possible neglect or misjudgment on their part or on the part of others. Self-blame was a common reaction, if parents felt that they did not do enough to protect the child. They may have become overwhelmed with guilt, chastising themselves for not having recognized the symptoms as polio, and not having acted sooner. Many survivors, in fact, wonder why their parents delayed getting them to a doctor—a nagging question that even today forms the basis of anger toward parents.

Since the symptoms of polio (fever, aches, pains) resembled those of minor ailments, many parents initially treated these complaints as just that—nothing out of the ordinary. The child was just not feeling well, the flu perhaps. Sometimes parents would even remember an incident that might have contributed to the symptoms: Tommy was around Uncle Bob who had a cold. Sara played jump rope too much last week; that's why she has pains in her legs. Mary is just trying to get out of school or trying to get attention.

But when the condition persisted and got even worse, parents had to consider that something else was going on. In such situations people move in and out of considering the possibility that something more serious is going on. It is hard to give up the sense of security that everything is familiar and under your control.

Acceptance of the Diagnosis

How quickly someone might have considered the culprit to be polio depended upon many factors. One was how much information they had about the disease. Although there were many articles in the press about polio, people's understanding of the details of the illness varied. Like any disaster, it always happened to someone else.

Eventually parents would take the child to the doctor, who most likely would have the child hospitalized. Parents were often kept in a state of ambiguity, as physicians did not always communicate a firm diagnosis at first. Giving "bad news" is very hard for many physicians, even today. And in those days physicians did not reveal everything to patients or their families.

Physicians might relay information bit by bit, thinking that the parents would gradually come to accept the diagnosis. However, parents would take every qualification as a sign that the diagnosis would turn out to be something other than polio. It was a paternalistic approach on the part of physicians that was supposed to protect patients and their family members—letting them have hope by withholding information that would frighten or upset them.

Over time, parents would vacillate between accepting that their child had polio to hoping that the doctors had made a mistake and would tell them so. At some point, however, the parents would finally accept the diagnosis, leaving them filled with feelings of helplessness and loss.

Later Adjustments

Those parents who after the first shock, managed to adjust, often did so by not excessively sympathizing or overprotecting their children. Although they were supportive, they focused on helping their children develop to their own potential.

AND NOW?

As mentioned earlier, some polio survivors still feel anger at their parents for not having identified the polio symptoms sooner. *"Perhaps I could have been treated more quickly and had a better recovery,"* a man tells me solemnly. However, as we see, the symptoms were not always that clear, and many parents had difficulty realizing that their child's condition was so serious.

Not being able to protect, care for, or visit their child during the treatment for polio was an ongoing emotional strain for many families. Sometimes treatment and rehabilitation took place far from home. Work demands or household duties would limit the time they had to visit.

A parent's not visiting the hospital or convalescent home would be experienced as abandonment by the child, but could have been related to many factors in addition to those above:

- A father's sense of powerlessness and lack of control might cause him to make excuses and avoid making the trip to visit his ailing child.

- A mother's being pulled between spending time with the ill child and taking care of other children at home might cause her to visit less than she would like.

Sometimes parents would feel detached, as though they were outside their bodies observing from a distance what was happening (a defense called dissociation, not unlike what many patients with polio experienced during their illness). Everything they did felt very mechanical; feelings were numb. Later parents may have felt ashamed that they had not cared for their child properly, feeling responsible for having allowed a child to become ill with this dreaded disease.

Certainly parents had a host of reasons for not being available for their sick child—some unavoidable and others related to resistance and denial. Unfortunately, there were few psychological and social services available for children and families in those days as compared to today.

Polio was an illness that affected (and affects) the entire family: parents, brother, sisters, grandparents. It was not an easy time for anyone.

However, many, if not most, survivors have good memories of a supportive home-life, and of loving, caring parents, who encouraged and helped them throughout their lives. This does not mean that at the same time they could not have conflicted feelings about their parents and the past. Although some parents may not have done the "right" things, most did the best they could to cope in these very difficult times.

YOUR AGING PARENTS

Some of you have parents who are still alive and need more attention than before. This comes at a time when you too are having more difficulties, with PPS, age-related illnesses, and other problems. You may find yourself reassuring your aging parents, even though you may be in need of reassurance yourself. This role reversal comes at a time when you may not be able to do as much as you used to; you wonder how you can do more for others when you cannot even do what you used to for yourself.

> *"How do I explain to my mother that I am no longer able to take care of her as I once did?"*

> *"How can I make my father understand that I get tired and don't have the stamina or strength I once had?"*

Martha, a polio survivor, has a mother who has always been a bit demanding, but it hadn't mattered so much over the years. Martha had a lot of energy and always found time to help her mother with her shopping and house cleaning. Now her mother is asking for more and more from Martha. Added to this is that her mother does not want to hear that her daughter doesn't always feel up to it.

"My mother gets upset if I try to tell her about the late effects of polio. She'll get angry and tell me that she's older than I am. How could I possibly have less energy than she has? Sometimes I think she hasn't gotten over the guilt that she has felt all these years—her guilty feelings that my polio was her fault. In the past she always was a bit self-centered and demanding. Now it's worse and becoming increasingly so as she ages. We fight all the time. She's even embarrassed when I use a brace or a cane."

Martha's mother appears to be having difficulty accepting what is happening to her and to her daughter, and acts as though her daughter's problems do not exist. Her mother is probably quite frightened, as she is struggling with her own dependency needs. She maybe asking herself (subconsciously):

"Who will take care of me? Who will take care of the two of us?"

This unwillingness to accept the realities of what is happening can cause great stress. Martha experiences it as her mother's not loving her anymore, not caring for her. With the advent of PPS, not only is the "child" revisiting polio, but the parent too is being forced to face those issues once again.

DEALING WITH PARENTS— NOW THAT YOU ARE A GROWN-UP

In day-to-day living you need to develop some coping skills to get by, when dealing with the issues related to your own parents and PPS. This is true whether they are still living or have passed on years ago.

- Understand that there most likely are complicated reasons behind your parent's behavior, today and in the past.

If your parent or parents are still living:

- Be realistic about what you can do for yourself and others.
- Set limits on how much you will do.

  You have a right to say no. You can do this pleasantly yet firmly. Be consistent so that the other person understands the message and is not confused.

- Ask for help from others if need be.
- Try to explain what is happening to you regarding PPS.
- Let your mother or father know that you are not deserting her or him, and that you will find others who will help with things that you have difficulty doing.
- Thank your parents and tell them you appreciate what they have done for you.
- Realize that the time to learn about what happened may be past; you may have to accept that and move on.

COMMUNICATION: NOTES OF CAUTION

Discuss polio and PPS with your aged parents only if you feel they are able to do so psychologically and physically. Pushing the subject of polio with elderly parents may only sink them into depression and agitation.

If a parent wishes to talk, listen. Ask a minimum of questions, if at all. The late years are not necessarily the moment to make up for lost time. Sometimes, even if a parent seems eager to talk, he or she may become flooded with upsetting thoughts and memories later on.

Be aware of underlying resentments and angers. Repressed feelings may surface now that roles are reversed and you are taking care of an aging parent.

If you harbor anger at your parents for past neglect or other reasons, there may be a conscious or unconscious wanting to punish them. One way to do this is to make them feel bad by going over your resentments or pointing out their faults. Even having them talk about the past when it is obviously upsetting may be a way to punish someone.

Taking advantage of a person's vulnerabilities, particularly when they are old and defenseless is no way to have healthy closure in your own life. And morally it is probably quite questionable.

A FINAL WORD

If your parents are no longer alive, try to let go. There is so much you don't know and will never know. Be careful in judging others. Life is not always what it seems, to quote an old adage.

There is not much you can do now about the negative, except work on your own thoughts and feelings. Focus on the positive aspects of what happened, or at least of what you remember. Take what lessons and what good you got from your parents and use it in the here and now.

14

SPOUSES AND
OTHERS SPEAK OUT

In a small study that I conducted about reactions to post-polio syndrome (PPS), I not only surveyed polio survivors, but also those who had accompanied them to the support group meeting. This group was mostly comprised of spouses, as well as a few brothers and sisters.

Granted those at the meeting were most likely people who were more understanding of PPS, but what they shared with me nevertheless gave insight into their internal struggles.

FAMILY MEMBERS: FEARS AND FRUSTRATIONS

Generally the significant others accepted their role as helper and felt important and useful. Their main complaint was "feeling low".

Many of the activities they used to enjoy doing with the survivor were no longer an option—activities such as dancing, skiing, and or sometimes even simply taking walks. They also missed doing things on their own. But given their new helping role, they felt they did not have the time for their own interests.

Some significant others found that over time the caretaking responsibilities were becoming more difficult for them, and they felt bad that they could not help the person with PPS, as they once did. They complained that the person with PPS was doing too much, and they wished they could be more helpful. But in some cases, the caretakers were having their own problems with aging, for example, some had developed illnesses of their own that complicated the situation.

These significant others reported having less energy and being less active than before. When they spoke of their own fatigue, they did so in an almost apologetic way—not being sure of how to deal with their own needs.

Overall, they felt frustrated and fearful and wished that they could change the situation.

GENDER DIFFERENCES IN EXPERIENCE AND EXPRESSION

Typically males and females differ in the way they express their feelings, both in words and behavior. This may be related to differences in the way men and women actually experience change and stress, or this may reflect socially-reinforced differences in how they have learned to express their feelings. For example, when men are depressed they may complain of physical ailments, whereas, women are more comfortable than men in talking about feelings and emotional difficulties.

In the polio-support group study, wives of polio survivors saw themselves as patient, but more anxious and depressed than they had been before their partner's PPS occurred. Some saw their spouses as understanding, while others reported increased tension and conflict at home.

Husbands of survivors reported being more irritable, more excitable, and feeling less optimistic than they had been in the past. They expressed frustration that their wives, who were experiencing PPS, often made it difficult for them to provide help, as they'd like to.

POSITIVE CARETAKING

At times, family members ask: "What about me?"

Caretakers need to stay healthy in mind and body. They need a break from the daily routine and demands and to take time for themselves. Yet these needs can cause internal conflicts, as significant others recognize that polio survivors cannot take a break from PPS. They feel guilty for thinking about their own welfare and pleasure.

Although family members may feel selfish doing something for themselves, if they get sick from stress, they will be of little help to those who need them. As much as possible, caretakers need to make room for their own lives. This is important for their mental health and may also be necessary for the family's financial well-being.

Balancing Needs and Interests

For family members, it is very important to have a life that includes others outside the family circle. Caretakers need to develop interests besides caretaking and household chores to help them relax and feel like a whole person. A positive mind and body is important for doing a better job in the care-taking role.

There are only so many hours in the day, but if we allocate them properly, we can often find some extra time for ourselves. Be flexible and adaptable. Find new interests compatible with the new life style.

POLIO SURVIVORS' VIEWS OF THEIR SIGNIFICANT OTHERS

Though the significant others have their own perspectives on the situation, these are not always understood or appreciated by those with PPS, who have their own competing fears and frustrations.

Survivors fear what the future holds. They are afraid of becoming a burden. They fear that they will place overwhelming demands on the family, and that family members will become resentful and withdraw.

Common complaints of those with PPS are that spouses often do not understand their frustrations and their fatigue:

> *"Sometimes he seems to 'forget', or he sees me as I was—not as I am."*

They also complain that family members often "do not seem to get it":

> *"My sister doesn't realize how tired I get and how much I cannot comfortably do now, in comparison to what I was able to do ten years ago."*

Being expected to do more than you feel you can do is an ongoing source of stress for the person with PPS and adds to feelings of guilt. But then, on the other hand, some polio survivors have the opposite problem: They feel that their family is "too protective."

The struggles between dependency and the desire to remain independent put conflicting strains on each party.

NEGATIVE BEHAVIORS: REAL OR PERCEIVED

Survivors complaints about their significant others cover the gamut. Family members are seen as over-protective, taking over, and paternalistic. They are described as angry and irritable, which some significant others admit to being. They wish their significant others would talk more about the PPS issues. They feel that when their requests are not met in a timely manner that means that the significant other does not remember that they have new PPS problems.

These are the perceptions of the polio survivors. Of course there is always the other side, as we have discussed.

GUIDELINES:
IMPROVING INTERPERSONAL RELATIONSHIPS

Following are some suggestions for both significant others and those with PPS.

Learn to

> Identify With The Other,
>   And
> Identify The Other's Needs.

It is not always easy at first to put yourself in someone else's shoes, particularly when you are fatigued, scared and possibly angry. But you need to work in tandem with the others in your home, if your own needs are to be met. And they won't be well met if your household is filled with tension. This is true if you are the polio survivor or the significant other.

So take the time, think in detail about the significant others in your life for a few minutes. Ask yourself:

- What might they be thinking now? Positive and Negative
- What are their interests? Strengths?
- What might they be thinking of me? Positive and Negative
- What might they be worried about?
- Do they have any personal needs that I am not noticing?
- What are their basic personality traits, and how can I work around them? For example,

     Is the person a procrastinator?

     Is the person easily angered?

- What makes them angry, anxious?
- What annoys me and how can I get around that?

And perhaps most importantly:

- What do I like about them?

Reread the list above, and make yourself write down answers to the questions. Don't just skim it, but take a paper and pencil now and really give these important items some concrete thought. It is not an easy task, but will help you negotiate your relationships with the significant others in your life.

COMMUNICATION: A TWO-WAY STREET

The subject of communication appears throughout this book, as it is extremely important for coping with PPS. Both survivors and significant others have thoughts and expectations that need to be communicated to each other, yet expressing them is not easy to do.

Survivors Speak Out

Survivors' biggest complaint is that others do not appreciate that they now have a more limited reserve of energy. Those with PPS may look the same as before, but that is not the case. PPS, particularly in the early phase, is one of those hidden conditions.

When asked what they would like family members to remember, the common responses are:

> *"When I say I'm tired, I mean it."*
> *and*
> *"Don't overestimate what I can do."*

These pleas translate into,

> *"Don't coax me to do something when I say I can't."*

Significant Others Speak Out

Family members also have their gripes. They would like to tell the survivors:

> *"Consider me too."*

> *"When you see I'm busy, give me time to finish what I am doing."*

> *"Thank me once in a while."*

LEARNING TO COMMUNICATE

You would think that it would be easy just to say what you feel to each other, but unfortunately life doesn't always work that way. If your needs are expressed during a heated exchange, they can be seen as self-centered. Much depends upon the tone of voice and when something is said. If people feel criticized, they get defensive and can respond angrily, without absorbing what is actually being asked of them. Each side feels not listened to, forgotten in the big picture.

Wait until things have cooled down. Work what you have to say into a conversation at a later time, where you will be able to explain how you feel and how the other person's behavior makes you feel. Notice that I am using the expression: "you feel", because all you actually know are your own feelings and thoughts. You really can't get inside the other person's head no matter how well you think you know them.

Don't tell your spouse that you think he doesn't care about you any more or that he only thinks of himself. Avoid attributing motivation to another person's behavior, as you may be wrong and then all you will get in response is resistance and anger.

NEGATIVE STATEMENT:

"I asked you six times, but you don't listen to me; you don't care."

Instead tell the other how certain specific behaviors affect your feelings.

POSITIVE STATEMENT:

"When you don't respond when I ask for something, it makes me feel sad and alone—that you don't care about me anymore."

Phrase yourself in terms of your own feelings, not what you think the other person is thinking and feeling. Let the person know how his or her behavior affects you, how it makes you feel. This approach allows room for dialogue as the other can tell you if you are right or not. He can explain himself, apologize, or tell you what you do that annoys him. Hopefully, if done in the right tone and if each side has a chance to speak, resentments can be minimized and each side learns to respect the other's needs.

This is not to say that there will not be miscommunications and arguments at times in families. Life has its stress and the vicissitudes of PPS add to the strife. By learning to talk to one another you can minimize these unpleasant interchanges and bring people closer together through understanding.

If trying these communication techniques on your own doesn't work, family therapy or counseling is a good place to go for help. This does not have to be a long-term commitment. A consultation with a professional sometimes is enough to help break through a communication barrier. Sometimes a few consultations spaced over several weeks or months are helpful to get feedback and make role and communication adjustments as needed.

SHARING INFORMATION ON PPS

Significant others need information to help them understand what is happening. They may not be able to absorb what they are being told due to their own anxieties about what is happening. Sometimes giving a little information at a time is the best way to proceed. Repetition is often necessary.

Written information is good, as it can be referred to later, and can be read and reread. Written information can also help alleviate misunderstanding. But be careful not to overload people with lengthy articles.

But, you say, no one in my family will read the information that I give them about PPS. Unfortunately many do not read what is given to them. Over time many who are at first resistant will take a peek at what is lying around and may eventually look at it. Be patient.

Table 3
FAMILY AND SURVIVORS SPEAK OUT

FAMILY MEMBERS' FEARS AND FRUSTRATIONS

Can't change the situation
Seeing the person with PPS doing too much
Seeing the person with PPS being in pain
Can't do what they would like to be doing themselves
Experiencing losses
> Can't do what used to do together
> Loss of control

SURVIVORS' FEARS AND FRUSTRATIONS

Afraid of what the future holds
Hate being judged by their appearance
Afraid of becoming a burden
> Needs will place overwhelming demands on family
> Fear family will become resentful and withdraw

FAMILY MEMBERS' NEGATIVE BEHAVIORS: REAL OR PERCEIVED

Over-protective
Take-over (give too much help)
Paternalistic (too much empathy)
Angry or irritable
Avoid talking about issues
Ignore requests
Forget have new PPS problems

Table 4

COMMUNICATING WITH SIGNIFICANT OTHERS

SURVIVORS SAY:

"When I say I'm tired, I mean it."

"Don't overestimate what I can do."

SIGNIFICANT OTHERS SAY:

"Consider me too."

"When you see I'm busy, give me time to finish what I am doing."

"Thank me once in a while."

◆   ◆   ◆

POSITITVE BEHAVIORS:

Think about what you really want, and how you can make it happen

...in a positive way.

Table 5

SIGNIFICANT OTHERS: GETTING A BALANCE IN YOUR LIFE

1. Plan for possible changes.
   Confront fears; develop a "just-in-case" attitude

2. Be flexible and adaptable.
   Find new interests compatible with your new life style, as needed.

3. Take time for yourself.

4. Have outside interests.

5. Develop a support network for socializing and for having more help.

6. Communicate. Talk to each other.

7. Do what you can to stay healthy physically and mentally.

8. Consider counseling or psychotherapy to help you:
   —Come to a comfortable stage of acceptance.
   —Integrate new and changing roles.
   —Improve communication, i.e., learn how to express feelings and needs.
   —Reduce chaos in the family or with friends.
   —Learn how to deal with others' fears and personalities and needs.

15

FRIENDS AND ACQUAINTANCES

Although friends can be included within the rubric of "significant others", I would like to devote a separate discussion to friends, as their importance in a person's life is often undervalued. Sometimes when people become ill or when they die, family members gather round and forget to notify or include close friends. Yet in all walks of life friendship plays a significant role—sometimes even more important than family. As the old adage goes: You choose your friends, but not your family.

Indeed, spouses are often described as dismissive, and children or siblings as not understanding or supportive enough. Friends, on the other hand, can be both understanding and supportive, and are often the ones who hear your deepest secrets. Networks of friends can be very helpful when you need to coordinate parts of your care. And they don't come with a lot of the family "baggage".

However, friends have their own lives and problems that need their attention, and some are better than others when it comes to being of help. Friends are usually not around as much as family, and thus, provide help in different ways. A difficulty that comes as one ages is that friends die, or they too become less able to do what they once did. They may be consumed by their own health issues or those of their own family members, and at times seem to disappear.

Nevertheless, do not underestimate the role and importance of friendship, particularly when you need help.

LIVING ON YOUR OWN

Friends are not given enough recognition for the supportive roles they play. Sometimes people who live alone and rely on friends actually have an easier time getting help when they need it, than do those who depend upon their spouse or children.

However, when you live alone, having post-polio syndrome (PPS) can complicate your life in different ways. You may have to hire people to do things for you, and that can be costly. You may try to avoid asking friends for help, as you see that they are busy with their own lives. Yet friends often jump to the cause when they can.

I have heard physicians referring to people who aren't married in ways that makes them sound as though they are all alone in this world. Yet I have seen friends stepping in to help in big ways, when someone is ill or in need.

I remember one such case when a physician referred a single woman to me who had cancer. He told me that she was all alone in the world and had no one to help her. But what I discovered was that she had a large network of very close friends, who were there in help her throughout her illness.

On the other hand, another woman, a widow whom I saw in my practice, had two grown children, who were somewhat estranged from her. She did have a demanding personality, and they tended to shy away from her even before her illness. When I first met the family, the son said to me with a sense of forewarning: "Good luck." Yet the physician thought the patient was well taken care of by her family. So you never know.

FRIENDSHIP: FINDING YOUR WAY

Perhaps you feel embarrassed and self-conscious around your friends, now that PPS has set in. The feeling of "not-wanting-to-be-a-burden" may make you pull back.

It may not be as easy visit with friends, since you can't get around as easily as you used to. You, thus, may find yourself increasingly isolated.

Also, if you have a friend who asks too many questions, you may find yourself avoiding that person. Sometimes you don't want to talk about what is going on, and would prefer friends just to act as diversions. There is something to be said for diversions, when you are not feeling well or are worried.

There is also something to be said for having someone lend you an ear for your woes, or having someone there who can help you find ways to make your life more comfortable. Friends can be valuable resources. It is getting that happy balance that is important.

Neighbors can be helpful too, should you be having trouble getting around. If you have a good relationship with your neighbors, they may be able to run some errands, since they have to come back to your neighborhood anyway. Even if you have family to help you, friends and neighbors can take up much of the slack. Divide your requests over several people, that way you won't become a burden, as you fear.

But remember friendship is a two-way street. It is something that needs to be nurtured over time Being demanding or whiney will not bring people to you. When you are isolated from others, you may talk too much to those who do come around. That is something to be watchful of and to avoid. Also, focusing too much on your own needs will not make people want to be with you for long.

Being kind and showing your appreciation is what bonds people together. Think of what you can do for others and what you can give to your friends. You may think that, since you are not feeling well, you have nothing to offer. But that is rarely the case. Start with "Thank you," and then think creatively.

By and large, for both the survivor and the survivors' family members, a circle of friends is an important resource for better health and a better quality of life.

16

DEVELOPING NEW RELATIONSHIPS

CONFRONTING FEARS

Sometimes new relationships make you get in touch with being disabled. They break down your defenses. That is why it may be hard to meet new people or to find yourself in unfamiliar situations.

Gloria has a lot of worries about new relationships. She had been married for 20 years, and now that she is divorced meeting new people and going places with them just fills her with apprehension. It doesn't matter if it's a date with a man, lunch with a new woman friend, or talking with a couple she's just met.

If she's invited to the theater, for example, she worries if there is a banister to hold onto, as she goes up the stairs. She wonders if the new friend will take her hand if she needs steadying. Before she ventures out she worries about everything.

"Will I be liked?"
"Will I make a fool of myself?"
"Will I sound stupid?"
"Will I look attractive?"
"Will I be rejected?"

"Will they be disgusted?"
"How will I explain my limitations?"
"Will I be helped if I need help?"

She foresees so many disasters that she often just postpones going out.

THE FACE

Gloria also feels that she has to present *the face*. One face she presents is: I can do it. She is one of those who have great difficulty asking for help. In her case, she is afraid of disappointing, of drawing attention, even of being abandoned.

She attributes this to her relationship with her mother when she was young. Her mother always focused on her own feelings, and when Gloria had any difficulties, like being teased in the schoolyard, her mother would say: "I feel so bad," putting her own emotions at the center.

"As a kid, I didn't want to upset my mother, so I didn't tell her anything bad that happened to me. I had to present 'the face', and I can still do it."

To this day, this protective and self-protective pattern has carried over into new relationships—interactions where Gloria still feels she has to put on *the face*. But it also means that she does not know how to be herself with others.

The face had other meanings for Gloria as well. She was always very pretty. She used her pretty face to keep people from focusing on her body and on her disability. She wore makeup perfectly and always wore her hair in a dramatic fashion.

Gloria was always looking at others, comparing herself to them. As she grew older, this became an obsession, and she began to panic: The white hairs, the lines, the skin losing it tightness and glow. She thought of a face-lift. But whatever she did she knew she couldn't be young again. Her face was failing her.

BODY IMAGE AND SELF-CONSCIOUSNESS

Rita, a widowed polio survivor in her 60's, would like to meet a man to share her life. Sal, her husband, had been a good support and friend throughout their long marriage. But Rita is reluctant to try to "get out there" and find someone new. Quietly she confides, *"Most men don't feel comfortable with a disabled person. It's hard to find one who accepts you."*

She fears things happening that could lead to *humiliation*: such as, her falling down, his noticing how awkwardly she walks. In thinking of an intimate relationship, Rita remembers how hard it was to date in high school: *"I just didn't dance right."*

Rita has become very self-conscious. Her teenage son did not help her poor body image, when he once remarked, "I'm so disgusted and embarrassed with you at the beach." Rita was very hurt. It made her feel that others think the same way, but just don't say so. She asks herself: *"If I am so disgusting on the beach, what about in the bedroom?"*

Women are not alone in worrying about new relationships and being concerned with their bodies. Harold had been teased as a child about his limp. The effects of the teasing stayed with him into adulthood, causing him to avoid new situations and acting aloof when he would meet people. He feared ridicule and rejection, and felt it was just better to be alone. In addition, his family still gives out confusing signals.

"I don't get much support or understanding from my family. They try to make me feel good by saying 'it's just a limp.' But it is more than 'just a limp.' It affects my whole life. Sometimes I think it defines who I am.

"I don't think they respect me and my struggle. My family never validated what I was going through, so I never did. I just suppressed my feelings. To this day my brother never asks how I am doing. If I try to talk about the late effects of polio he just changes the subject. I don't know if this is a lack of interest or his discomfort. Whatever it is, it affects the way I see myself. Sometimes I wish I could just hide."

MALADAPTIVE DEFENSES IN SOCIAL RELATIONSHIPS

So how do your psychological defenses play out in regard to others, particularly those whom you wish to impress?

Withdrawal

Some people defend themselves from the pain of social rejection by withdrawing from others. As one woman describes this:

"I find myself falling out of love with friends."

By this she means that she becomes more critical of others, which provides a rationale for the withdrawal.

Denial

Some survivors deny even wanting or needing a relationship in their life. They can give you a litany of reasons why. And maybe they are right. But in many cases they use denial to guard against the hurt that comes from friendships that don't work out.

As part of this denial, they act very independent and send out the message: *"Don't come near, don't help me."* What they are really saying inside is *"Don't make me love you. I may get hurt."*

Avoidance

Related to the defense of withdrawal is avoidance, in this case the avoidance of having relationships. What one is really trying to avoid is rejection. Like Harold, some survivors have a history of being teased at school—others, of not being wanted in the family. They fear facing that hurt again.

Bill remembers how he and his sister used to walk to school together. They were sweet memories for him, until one day, not long ago, when they were both well into adulthood. His sister, in this age of "letting-everything-out", told him how she hates walking with him because he is so slow. She went on to admit that she used to feel "stuck with him" when they walked to school in those years passed.

Bill's sweet memories were crushed.

When Bill told her how much it hurt to hear that, his sister replied: *"It's good I can be honest."*

The so-called honesty did not cushion Bill's hurt. It only served to reinforce his fears that people have disdain for him. *"It is like a sting,"* he says. *"You know someone and then something happens: your siblings, your kids, your parents, your spouse. With new people it's even worse; you're afraid to take a chance, afraid of being hurt again. You don't want to be "put-up-with or tolerated; you want to be really accepted."*

AVOIDING THE TRAPS

You may feel needy, even desperate for new friends or a new relationship. This can make you vulnerable and cause you to do or say things that later you may regret. Feeling needy or desperate can make you talk too much, try too hard. This drives people away.

- Take your time.
- Think things through.
- Think about what you want and who you are.

Because of past experiences, you may not know how to show your feelings: deep inside is a mixture of sadness and anger. You fear that if you show your feelings and your neediness, you won't be loved; you'll be abandoned. You've learned over the years to keep things to yourself. Thus, you don't know how to let others know who you really are.

Some people feel that they are basically bad, and if others get to know the real them they would be shocked. This negative self-image is often a result of traumatic experiences from childhood. They feel that they are not worthy of love. This can happen if you were criticized a lot and told you were bad, or if you were abused as a child. Such traumatic events happened in patients' polio experiences but are not readily talked about.

You internalize the words and the associated feelings, and it is very difficult to get rid of them as you grow up. If you were told you were bad at an impressionable age, the idea of yourself as not worthy or acceptable stays with you. Thus, you have the additional fear that those you meet will learn your secrets and then abandon you because of them. Or worse, they may turn out to be as bad as those you trusted years ago who turned on you.

In terms of your own conflicts about who you are, it is not necessary to let people know whom you think you are deep down inside. You don't have to share all with everyone. Some people will get to know one side, and some another. That is the nature of relationships. But first you must learn to accept yourself.

As time goes on and relationships develop, people will discover things about you gradually. The foundation of the relationship will determine how much the other person wants to know and needs to know—and how much you are willing to share about yourself.

ACCEPTING YOURSELF

Learning to accept yourself takes time and, believe it or not, practice. At first you may have to pretend or act in ways that do not feel natural. You may have developed a persona that included thoughts and behaviors that kept people at bay. You now have to be like an actor and practice being the someone you would like to be—and that someone is probably who you really are but have hidden for so long.

As part of this new approach to forming new relationships, you will find yourself talking more to others and venturing out more. Study the following table for tips on how to handle meeting people and being in new situations.

Table 6

BEING YOURSELF IN RELATIONSHIPS

SELF-CONSCIOUSNESS
Accept who you are and who you can be.
Let go of past images and create a new self.

PREPARATION
Imagine new situations and how you'd like to act.
Role-play in your mind.

CONVERSATION
Smile. Make eye contact.
Monitor how much you talk about yourself.
Ask others about themselves.
Observe boundaries: others and your own.

THE TRAPS
Feeling needy and desperate.
Fear of rejection: Don't "over-worry" about rejection.
Personalization:
   Don't relate everything to yourself:
   People have their own issues, and their reactions
   may have nothing to do with you.

Positive Actions
Reframing: Change negative thoughts to positive ones.
Monitor anger.

MEDICAL CARE

17

PATIENT-DOCTOR RELATIONSHIPS

SURVIVORS SPEAK OUT ABOUT DOCTORS

Those who are experiencing the late effects of polio are quite frustrated with the lack of knowledge on the part of most physicians about polio and post-polio syndrome (PPS). They feel that some doctors are in "disbelief" when they, the patient, suggest PPS as possibly underlying their symptoms.

"Doctors do not understand what we are going through. They have not studied about polio, much less PPS."

"Family physicians do not understand PPS and some don't even try—and that includes orthopedic specialists in some cases."

"They are unfamiliar with PPS, and in particular pulmonary complications. Also, they don't understand how other conditions, like menopause, are affected by PPS."

"My family physician diagnosed me as being "clinically depressed" two years ago. He did not believe PPS really existed."

One woman said that her physician was a pleasant man, but she did not believe that he read the post-polio literature she gave him. A male survivor confided to me in the same vein:

"I have difficulty getting physicians to listen to me and to try new things.

"Some of them are really thick. They think they know everything when they don't really know what is going on. What makes me angry is when I try to explain something, and they patronize me."

And another man, who was looking for an evaluation and diagnosis for his new symptoms, said with a sense of weariness:

"I have never been diagnosed with PPS, but I believe that I am beginning to experience symptoms of PPS. I am seeing physicians for various ailments that they can't diagnose. I just don't know whether I have post-polio syndrome or not."

DIAGNOSING PPS

As a result of the success of the polio vaccines, few physicians today have had training or experience in treating polio patients. Many are unaware of PPS, leaving patients disappointed and scared as they search for help.

Misdiagnosis is not uncommon; for example, in some cases patients with PPS have initially been diagnosed as having Amyotrophic Lateral Sclerosis (ALS—Lou Gehrig disease) because of the similarity of symptoms.

Many polio survivors (particularly those with milder impairments) have avoided medical specialists for years, either not needing care or having had their fill of it. Now when faced with PPS symptoms and other conditions associated with aging, they soon become aware that those they must turn to for help are operating in a new area and are not always sure what to do.

RESISTANCE TO TREATMENT

Compounding the emergence of PPS is that survivors have been told that the very treatment used years ago (e.g., to exercise as much as possible) may have exacerbated the present condition. Today polio survivors are being told to take it easy, not to over-do it, to rest more, and to accept the lessening strength and stamina.

Logically this advice may make sense, but emotionally such changes in life style are difficult to achieve, particularly when former patients have spent a lifetime believing what they were doing was good for them. Resistance to change is a natural reaction, but in this situation, even more resistance occurs since individuals are advised to curtail many pleasure s and become more dependent on others.

In addition, hope may be shattered and trust in authority shaken. Patients become aware that recent recommendations for treatment are based on new, relatively untested theory, as were many of the directives given years ago with such authority, that are now being questioned.

Thus, health care providers find patients avoiding treatment, minimizing their conditions, and disregarding advice—in effect, not wanting to curtail their activity, particularly when, in their minds, no one is really sure.

CONFLICTS BETWEEN PHYSICIAN AND PATIENT

Sometimes treatments or surgeries for PPS ailments or other medical conditions may not be as successful as hoped for by the survivor or the physician. Post-operative complications abound, because muscles may be too weak to give needed support, bones won't mend, and deterioration continues. Physicians, out of feelings of impotence and frustration, can become defensive, i.e., avoiding the patient and not answering questions.

Although the available literature encourages those with PPS to keep themselves informed, this same literature is filled with frightening prospects, making people anxious when going to medical appointments for fear of what they may be told. When questions are not answered directly, survivors can become angry since they feel that information is being withheld or that the doctor really doesn't know how to treat their condition.

DIFFERENT PERSONALITIES

In medicine these days, patients can't just lay back and let the doctors and nurses take total charge. Not only is it good for you to share information with the medical practitioners, but many times they try to engage you in the decision-making. You are informed of what is to happen, what your options are, and what you can expect. Sometimes the amount of information given to you is overwhelming in its detail or in the speed at which it is presented. This can put pressure on you, depending upon your personality make-up.

People differ in the ways that they manage information, in terms of how much information they can tolerate at any one time, and the extent to which they wish to be involved in the decision-making. For some, having information helps them to feel in control. When denied information about their condition, they become anxious and angry. They prefer to take an active role in their care.

Others do not want to know very much, and become quite anxious when given too much information too soon. They prefer to let the doctor make the decisions and prefer to be involved as little as possible.

You may recognize yourself as one of these personality types, or perhaps you fall somewhere in between. Figure out what your information tolerance level is, and then let your doctor know how much you want to be involved.

18

AVOIDING GOING TO THE DOCTOR

As a polio survivor, you may have had your fill of going to doctors, so you delay following up on health-related problems. However, with age, new medical conditions arise that need attention.

Physicians often wonder why patients wait so long before coming to see them. There are many reasons, which are tied to how people perceive their conditions, as well as their characteristic ways of handling anxiety, and their past experiences with illness and disability.

THE FEAR OF KNOWING

The fear of a "bad" diagnosis and concerns about treatment can strongly influence the decision to put off a visit to the doctor. Yet with some medical conditions, acting in a timely manner takes care of a problem that could only get worse. A delay may, in effect, lead to the feared extensive treatment, the feared pain, and the feared disability. Although most people know this intellectually, putting off going to the doctor is a common occurrence.

Some people wonder if the doctor will consider them to be hypochondriac, vain, or someone who is wasting their precious time. They say to themselves:

"Maybe it's in my mind."
"Maybe it will go away."
"I'll go to the doctor later, when I have more time."

Often these thoughts are just rationalizations that help you to procrastinate even more.

FAMILY AND FRIENDS

Friends and family can be very supportive and urge you to seek evaluations or treatment, when you are in a hiding and avoiding mode. Invite one of them to come to appointments with you, in case your anxieties make you want to delay the visit. Also, you will then have four ears instead of two, in case the anxieties interfere with your listening and understanding all that goes on in the doctor's office.

But bear in mind family and friends have their own personalities and coping strategies. They also have their own limits regarding how much they can take on, both practically and emotionally. Since these people are not acting as professionals, they may inadvertently add to the problem.

In trying to alleviate anxiety—yours and their own—significant others may say, "Don't overreact", and thus add to the denial. Or the contrary, their persistent urging that you see a physician may set up more resistance on your part. But overall try to be open to their support and use it wisely.

HIDDEN WORRIES

As a patient you may be worried about things that your doctor has not even considered?

"Will I suffer? Will I be in pain?"
"Can I afford it? Will my health insurance cover this?"
"Will I be incapacitated?"
"Will I be able to work during and after treatment?"
"How will I be able to take care of my family?"
"Will I be disfigured?"
"Am I going to die?"

These reasons or rationalizations are outlined in the following table, aptly called: *Reasons for Delaying Going to the Doctor.*

- Look closely at the list of reasons for delay.

- Check those that apply to you, and when possible discuss these issues with your physician.

- Search for solutions to those that are getting in the way of your seeking the care that you need.

Table 7

REASONS FOR DELAYING GOING TO THE DOCTOR

- Lack of accurate information about one's condition

- Procrastination—feeling that treatment is not urgent

- Wish to avoid the expense of medical treatment

- Responsibilities related to self, family, and work

- Other medical conditions given priority

- Memories of your own or others' illnesses

- Distrust of the physician's competence or skill

- Personal dislike of the physician

- Fear of pain and disfigurement

- Fear of finding out that one has a serious, perhaps fatal illness

- Normal coping mechanisms, such as denial, avoidance, and anger

- Underlying psychiatric disorder which interferes with perception and judgment

19

BEING PART OF THE TEAM

EDUCATING YOUR DOCTOR

Polio newsletters often have editorials urging those with the late effects of polio to educate their physicians about post-polio syndrome (PPS). Some polio survivors have expressed concern about doing this, wondering:

> *"Will doctors really listen to me?"*
> *"Will they get angry with me for trying to tell them what to do?"*
> *"Will I transmit the information correctly?"*

Patients have underlying fears about "educating" their doctors:

- A fear of making the doctor defensive — of having the doctor withdraw from them, yell at them, or criticize them.

- A fear of having a condition that is not well understood, and realizing the doctor doesn't know enough or doesn't care enough to learn.

Some survivors resent the idea of having to "educate" their doctors—saying that: "The doctor should know. I'm paying him; why should I be the one to tell him anything?"

Resentments come from wanting to be taken care of and then feeling that you are being asked to take care of the doctor, so to speak.

WHAT ABOUT SPECIALISTS?

Perhaps you say to yourself: "I'd prefer to go to a specialist; then I wouldn't have to do any educating." There are unfortunately at present no official medical specialties in PPS. But there are, however, physicians who have an interest in and experience in that area. Sometimes this comes about because the doctor has had polio, or someone in his or her family has had it. In other cases, polio survivors have appeared in physicians' practices and stirred their interest in PPS.

Trying to find a physician who is knowledgeable about PPS can be difficult, depending upon where you live. Your local support group may be able to help you find a knowledgeable doctor in your area.

TAKING AN ACTIVE ROLE IN YOUR HEALTHCARE

There is a flood of information on all kinds of medical problems and new information coming out every day. Physicians are very busy, they have many pressures on them, and there is only so much they can do to stay abreast in their fields. If they don't have many (or any) patients with PPS, they may not have had a reason to keep up with the literature or the latest developments related to polio. They may care, but not have the time or incentive to investigate the area.

Pointing physicians in the direction of your concerns by giving them condensed information on the subject is one way to go. But how to do this without offending anyone?

TECHNIQUES FOR IMPROVING COMMUNICATION

Begin with a positive attitude.

Approach physicians in a polite way, saying that you believe or have been told that you have PPS. Ask if they have had much experience treating people who have had polio. Tell them that you have some material with you and ask if they would like to have it. Show respect for their training and time.

Be concise and to the point.

Don't overload doctors with stacks of articles or articles that are overly long or say the same thing. Find something that illustrates what you feel is important to your case. They may not have the time to read lengthy articles, but they might appreciate something they can refer to, or something that will lead them to places where they can research on their own, such as web sites.

Think of yourself as being part of a team.

Not that you are on equal levels on all fronts, but it is your body and you all have something to gain through cooperation. How you deal with your physicians depends upon their personalities and your own. Try to find those with whom you feel comfortable—but primarily, physicians you feel are professional and willing to work as a team.

Come to the appointment prepared.

Write down a list of questions beforehand, so that you can clearly go over each one. You could even give a copy of your questions to your physician. Review the list before the visit. Revise it by prioritizing from most important to least. Make sure that it includes the most important questions and concerns.

20

A PHYSICIAN'S GUIDE: UNDERSTANDING POST-POLIO SYNDROME

A LACK OF TRUST

Physicians and other medical personnel need to be aware that polio survivors have had a lot of experience with the medical world. This has left many with a certain level of understanding, as well as a certain level of distrust for those in authority.

They have noticed the confusion on the part of physicians today in diagnosing and treating post-polio syndrome (PPS). Complicating matters, medical problems that come with aging are interacting with the late effects of polio, making diagnosis more difficult.

Having had prolonged hospitalizations in the past, polio survivors are now more aware of errors and foibles that can happen even with the best and latest medical care. Although they may not have known much about what was going on when they had polio as young children, now much is written about the earlier treatment and its limitations. Polio survivors realize that the physicians in the past, though well meaning, may have been misdirected or even wrong about diagnosis and treatment.

Some physicians are good listeners and may even read the literature brought to them by patients. But far too many are "busy" and don't have the time, or take the time, to understand post-polio syndrome. Some can become irritated if patients try to talk about PPS. They may also become quite defensive and angry, if they think patients know more (or think they know more) than the doctor does. Aware of this, many polio survivors are hesitant to bring their PPS concerns to physicians, feeling they may not be informed or sympathetic to their distress.

EARLY TREATMENT AND ITS AFTERMATH

Underlying the care that polio patients received years ago were treatment approaches that are questioned today and that had unexpected consequences.

Early Beliefs

One belief was that to get better you had to exercise—the more the better. This idea is now being questioned; thus adding to survivors' concerns about how much to believe of what they are told today. Some fear that all the exercise they did in the past has now exacerbated their symptoms.

Others speculate that with time PPS would have developed anyway, and that the early bouts of exercise gave people added strength and a better quality of life until now. In any event, the idea of doing a lot of exercise was a clinical judgment that was not necessarily based on scientific evidence. It was helpful at the time, but the long-term effects were not known.

Former Treatment

One needs to remember all that these young (and sometimes older) polio patents went through. It was not just the acute trauma but also the years of treatments and separation from family and friends.

It was common to splint and cast. Young people would lay in body casts for months. Psychologically this restriction of movement was especially hard for the young. There was also the possibility of physical damage and the atrophying of muscles leading to other difficulties.

Sister Kenny used warm moist heal (wool) packs in combination with early activity. She challenged the medical establishment and the idea of immobility. Now people even wonder if this form of treatment was the best way to go.

In the case of bulbar polio, tracheotomy was used in 50% of the cases on the West coast and 6% elsewhere—another trauma for those being treated: Where you lived determined your type of care.

Over the years there could be surgeries, depending on the person's condition: fixing joints, lengthening and shortening extremities, increasing articulation, transferring muscles. School age patients spent many summers in hospitals.

TREATMENT PROBLEMS TODAY

Treatment is not always successful—that was true for the past and is so for medical problems polio survivors have now.

Medical Complications

Physicians today may underestimate how weak polio survivors' muscles actually are. One woman had abdominal surgery that needed several repairs because her abdominal muscles were too weak—a side effect of the polio. In another case, a patient's back muscles were not strong enough to give support after back surgery, leading to much pain and several additional major surgeries.

Given these complications, physicians can become defensive and, in this day and age, worried about malpractice suits. They feel impotent and frustrated, and thus, avoid patients' questions.

Patients' Regressive Behaviors

Physicians may see patients with PPS exhibiting regressive behaviors, such as, resisting medical advice, taking risks, not going for tests, smoking, or asking endless questions. They may feel frustrated, thinking those patients are not taking care of themselves. Yet this behavior is often a patient's attempt, though maladaptive, to gain control over uncontrollable feelings and events.

RECOGNIZING PSYCHOLOGICAL DISTRESS

Physicians often make the argument that the medical concerns related to life and death come first, with psychological and quality-of-life issues a distant second. It is a strong argument.

Yet mental health professionals working with persons with illnesses and disabilities know how often quality-of-life issues come up and how important these issues are to patients' well-being, often affecting compliance with treatment. Physical pain and suffering are not the only suffering a person must endure.

There is also psychological-emotional pain. As with discomfort associated with physical illness, there are treatments to lessen psychological pain and suffering. To ignore or minimize the emotional components of medical conditions can be quite counterproductive to say the least.

Physicians need to understand that the patients experiencing the late effects of polio may be seeing themselves as disabled for the first time—even though these polio survivors may have had some residual weakness and mobility problems from the acute polio. This is indeed a new self-concept, and one that comes with a sense of loss, a change of roles, and a fear for what the future may bring.

MAKING REFERRALS

Using psychologists or other mental health professionals as part of the treatment team is important, since physicians often do not have the time nor training to deal with patients emotional needs.

Watch the Tone of Voice

Referrals for psychological help should be given in the same professional manner as referrals to a medical specialist—and not with an exasperated tone that suggests the patient is a bother. When making a referral, the physician should be aware of the way in which the referral is done. For some people there is still a stigma about seeing a therapist—a stigma unfortunately still shared by some physicians. The physician's own bias may show through in tone or choice of words.

One polio survivor was told that she was "fixated" on post-polio syndrome and needed to see a therapist. Though this was an appropriate referral, the tone that the physician used made the survivor feel that she was being dismissed. She also felt that the doctor was telling her accusingly:

"You should have your head examined."

In this case, the physician had picked up on her anxiety. This obsession or "fixation", as he called it, reflected an underlying fear that those with PPS have about their future. And related to this, her preoccupation with PPS also reflected her frustration in trying to manage her own care in this haphazard medical environment we have today.

The physician, who suggested that the patient see a therapist, should be commended; however, a different tone of voice may have helped the patient accept the referral and feel less dismissed. Many physicians do not recognize the emotional turmoil that those with PPS go through, trying to get good care and worrying about the future.

Toughing-It-Out

In addition, physicians are often amazed at the patient's ability to adapt to obvious disabilities, and commend the polio survivors for "toughing it out"—not recognizing their need for help. But some may need assistance in this "toughing-it-out"—a place to vent their angers and fears, to relieve stress, to get support, to find out how they are doing psychologically and how they can find a release for their tensions. By helping the patient deal with the psychological issues—by referring out if necessary, the physician can then focus on the medical needs.

Table 8

WORKING WITH PATIENTS WITH PPS: SUGGESTIONS FOR PHYSICIANS

1. Listen to your patients with PPS, as they know their bodies, past and present.
2. Be aware of your own reactions, so they will not get in the way of your relationship with your patient and compliance with treatment.
3. Read the literature that they give you on PPS. (If you are reading this material, you are probably the kind of physician who does read material that patients bring you.)
4. Reassure the patients with PPS that they do not have a new neurological disorder, such as ALS (assuming that this is so).
5. Consider having the patient do gentle exercises and pay attention to fatigue. Rest is important.
6. Use a treatment team approach
   a. Refer the patient, if necessary, to a physical therapist who has specific experience with PPS.
   b. Consider referrals to mental health professionals to help with adjustment issues and re-emerging issues from the past. And be sure to include the patient and the family as part of the treatment team.

MENTAL HEALTH

21

TACKLING STRESS

WHAT DO WE MEAN BY STRESS?

Stress: Mental, emotional, or physical strain caused, for example, by anxiety or overwork. Stress may cause symptoms, such as raised blood pressure or depression.

Stressful: Demanding, taxing, worrying, traumatic, tense, nerve-racking

Synonyms: Pressure, strain, anxiety, constant worry, tension

Stress comes in many forms.

- There are high stress and low stress situations.

- There are the annoyances, the everyday worries, and the more generalized fearful anxieties.

- There are times when you feel you can do something about what bothers you; and there are instances when you feel things are just not in your control.

When the situation feels out of control, stress can attack the body, lowering your resistance and making you susceptible to other difficulties, possibly even making you sick. However, when you feel that you can eventually make it through, that you can find some way to solve the problem, then there is less wear and tear on your body and your psyche, as well.

STRESSFUL EXPERIENCES IN EVERYDAY LIFE

Throughout this book we have examined polio survivors' psychological adjustments to post-polio syndrome (PPS). In this chapter we are looking at certain situations that polio survivors have identified, as annoyances, worries, and sources of stress in their everyday lives.

Getting Out and About

Just going to visit others or going to social events can feel overwhelming. Even very immediate and practical every day concerns can cause survivors to feel stress.

What to wear.   When going out, one concern is what to wear. For women with PPS one major hurdle is finding the right shoes. This may not sound like much, but for those with mobility problems finding suitable shoes can cause all kinds of stress. Some may discount such concerns as just vanity. But vanity should not be dismissed so easily, as it plays a very important role in how you feel about yourself: your self-respect and the respect you feel from others. Your ego is important; it affects the quality of your life.

> *Paula was quite concerned about how she'd look at her son's wedding. She always dreamed of wearing a lovely dress and walking down the aisle with style and grace. She didn't want to wear "sensible shoes". They would spoil her outfit; Heels would look the best, but they would also make her feel unstable and anxious. As it was she felt self-conscious about the way she walked.*

After a lot of looking Paula did manage to find a compromise pair of shoes—not too high, not too low, but the internal struggle before finding the solution was painful for her. She wanted to fit in. She wanted to have her dream.

What Paula finally did was to *compromise*. You may not like the word. You may get tired of compromising, but for stress reduction it has its place, as long as you don't dwell on the part that you have given up.

Weather concerns. When it's wet and cold, you may become afraid of falling, particularly if it is icy. Driving may also become a concern. This is true as people age, not only for those with PPS. However, with PPS the possibility of falling may be greater, as will the potential for hurting yourself and having a longer recovery time.

Doug cancels plans on occasion for fear of falling. What he hates most about that is having to explain why he isn't coming. "Others just don't understand," he complained to me. "They ask too many questions; they try to coax me. Sometimes I go, even when I don't want to, just to avoid the pressure from my friends."

Being with friends can help reduce life's stress, so maybe Doug is better off in the long run making the effort. However, worrying about getting there and back, and risking the possibility of an accident, may cancel out the benefits.

How to get a balance? Doug needs to get in touch with his feelings—to distinguish between when he is avoiding people because he feels frustrated and down, and when he really doesn't have a good way to get some place.

Accessibility—or lack thereof. On the list of most annoying things, polio survivors put lack of accessibility at the top. Not being able to get into theatres, public buildings, stores, and restaurants is very frustrating, often leading to a sense of injustice.

The lack of accessibility to bathrooms in public buildings and on airplanes is particularly stressful. Some public bathrooms claim to be handicapped accessible, but often you can't get in with a wheelchair, or can't maneuver properly once inside. The inconvenience and humiliation is sure to raise blood pressure and weigh on self-esteem.

One woman complained bitterly of having an "accident", because she was not able to attend to her *"bathroom functions in a timely manner."* A man told of his embarrassment because the toilet in the handicap bathroom was so low that he had to wait for help in order to get up. The grab bars were there, but they were too far away and too high to be of any use.

Even simple things become a worry, like wanting to go to the theatre but not knowing if there will be banisters to help navigate the stairs.

> *"And whose hand would I hold, if I need help?" Barbara asked. "My family often acts like they don't know me, when we are out in public. I think they are tired helping, or even a bit ashamed to this day. Sometimes it's just easier to stay home."*

Another area not often mentioned is the difficulty getting up and down the steps in other people's houses. The inability to visit friends on their turf puts a hidden strain on relationships. You may feel like you are bothering others when trying to figure out how to get inside a house safely. And you may feel that you are asking for special favors by always suggesting that you meet in a restaurant or at your home.

Where accessibility is concerned, there inevitably seems to be something that you have to be paying attention to. And of course one person's accessible space may be another person's barrier.

Vacations.   Going on a vacation is supposed to be relaxing. But as we all know that in today's world traveling can be very stressful for everyone. Just trying to plan the trip and negotiate taxis and airports are major hurdles for the twenty-first century traveler. For someone with special needs, it is even more complicated.

Getting onto airplanes, for example, is problematic. Although airlines try to make accommodations, there is no end to the worrisome stories of not being able to get on the plane, problems with wheelchairs, or being dropped by someone when being lifted—to name a few. Unfortunately you need to anticipate some of these problems when planning a trip.

Planning takes a lot of time and attention to detail to make sure that places and transport are accessible. Some find the Internet a useful place to get information. Talking to others in your support group, and reading support group newsletters are good ways to get some tips. And there is nothing like calling directly and making your requests by phone.

Surprises do await you nonetheless. You cannot always be sure that when you arrive somewhere your requests will be met. As you may have already experienced, those without special needs often think a place is accessible when in fact it is not. The hotel bed may be too high, or the room too cluttered for your chair to move around easily or at all.

The airline may not have a wheelchair ready even though you reserved one; or there may be a "small step or two" at the entrance to the restaurant that no one thought would be a problem. How many times have you heard: *We can carry you in*? Right! Talk about stress.

You need to make a list of your special needs and questions to help assure that you get what you want. Be specific. Going with a tour group that specializes in tours for people with disabilities may take some of the worry out of your vacation. But group travel isn't for everyone.

Peter, a survivor, explained to me that he and his wife go to the same place in Florida every year. This takes the guesswork out of much of the trip. But what he hates is that his wife has to do all the packing and unpacking, as he is unable to do so anymore. And she also has to do the heavy lifting of the suitcases along the way. This is a downer for him, as he used to be the strong one.

Cognitive Therapy Exercises: When in a situation like this, you need to reframe your thoughts from negative to positive; you need to change the way you talk to yourself. Peter should remind himself from time to time that his wife wants his company. Although she may prefer to have someone help her, she is probably happy to do what she can to make their winter stay possible. He must also remind himself that there are other things that he gives to her and does for her that help make her life pleasant and fulfilling.

Traveling with friends. Being on vacation with friends can be trying. As someone with PPS, you try to balance your needs with the group's activities.

If you move slowly, you may be concerned about holding other people up. As others try to see how they can accommodate you, you begin to feel that you are losing a certain sense of privacy. They ask questions in order to understand your needs, so you find yourself explaining when you'd rather not. As a result they learn more about your weaknesses and losses than you'd like them to know. At times your traveling companions may encourage you to do something, when you may not want to be encouraged. These concerns can weigh on your mind and interfere with the pleasure of your vacation.

Cognitive Therapy Exercises: Remember that traveling with others can be quite fun. It helps to know your traveling companions fairly well and to discuss with them your concerns before you go. Set limits to what you will discuss and what you are comfortable doing. Maintain your personal boundaries, and develop ways to do so politely while on the trip. Then try to let yourself enjoy your vacation.

Other Peoples' Responses

One area that causes stress is other peoples' responses to disability. Feeling that "people don't understand or look down on people with disabilities" can be very unsettling. What are they thinking? Why do they look at me? When they compliment me, can I take it seriously, or are they just patronizing me?

Anna has a different reaction when she is with others. She does not like to be the center of attention, as she feels she got so much attention as a child. People looking at her, or wanting to help her, all this makes her feel guilty—guilty for stealing attention away from her brother and sister when they were young.

Anna says she is "afraid of other people's jealousy", so she keeps a low profile and tries not to draw attention to herself. If she is given a promotion or is given something special, she fears the reactions of others. She wonders:

> *"Do they feel sorry for me? Do they think I'm odd? Do they really appreciate me? If they like me, I still feel guilty, since I got so much attention as a child. I wonder, maybe they will turn on me,"*

WORK-RELATED ISSUES AND RETIREMENT

Work, almost by definition, comes with stress. I guess that's why it is called work. For someone with a disability there is the added stress of wanting to do a good job, but not being able to function in an environment that may not be set-up completely for someone with different needs. And bosses who are demanding and not in tune with the needs of disabled people (despite ADA) can make life difficult.

More stress comes from within: from the pressure to achieve and be up there with the best. This ideal which many polio survivors have internalized has been laid at the feet of those early caregivers, who told those with polio to keep trying, to fit in, to be the best—and in some cases not just the best they can be, but the best. Now that's stress.

Retirement comes with its own stresses, as you may not be able to do all the things you planned to do when you quit working. What to do with your free time, now that you have this time on your hands? Being around family members all day can cause tension, as you interfere with their daily routines. These problems are common for many retirees, but are more complex for those with PPS, who may have more limited possibilities or find the solutions to their plans difficult to work out.

Cognitive Therapy Exercises: In trying to work out your new life style, see the process as part of life itself and a learning experience. Break down the issues into small steps that you can analyze and work on one by one.

MEDICAL PROBLEMS

One of the major complaints that survivors have is finding good physicians who are knowledgeable about PPS. Since polio has been almost completely eradicated in the world, physicians often come out of training with no experience or knowledge about polio and PPS. This is also true when it comes to physical therapists and mental health practitioners. (Other issues related to physicians and medical cares are covered in the chapter on Physicians.)

One of the most trying situations that polio survivors share with others is waiting for the results of medical tests, such as MRIs. The mind can lead you into worries of all kinds. Those who have had polio may find themselves having flashbacks or frightening memories from their past experiences with the medical profession, when they first had polio.

Cognitive Therapy Exercises: During these tense waiting-periods, which can go on for days or weeks, remind yourself that there is only so much you can do until you get the results. Do whatever you can to distract yourself from negative thoughts. Keep busy. Listen to music.

When you do find yourself worrying, force yourself to think of other more pleasant things:

- Think of yourself being with friends or family that you like.
- Dream about a vacation in the sun on a beautiful beach. Use your senses to feel the wind on your cheek and the sun on your face; imagine listening to the waves.
- Do a Thought-Stopping exercise:
- Simply repeat the words: Stop…Stop…Stop—over and over until you push those negative thoughts out of your head

These Relaxation and Stress Reduction techniques from Cognitive Therapy are easy to do at home—although like physical exercise they do take some practice.

MAJOR WORRIES

Aging and the Future

If you have PPS, you most likely have fears of what lies ahead. You are not alone in worrying about the future as you age. But your earlier experience with polio can heighten your anxiety.

Specifically, polio survivors have told me that they worry about:

- Isolation.

  "My children go on with their lives and don't spend as much time with me anymore. On top of it many of my friends have died or moved away."

- Dependency and being less able to take care of things as before.

  "I'm afraid of becoming dependent on others. What if my health deteriorated or my husband died. Who would take care of me?"

- Moving to a retirement home or nursing home, settings which bring back many memories from the past.

  "I'm afraid of losing the ability and energy to function by myself, of being unable to care for myself."

- Illness and injury leading to hospitalizations.

  "I worry about breaking a bone, my arm would be the worst, as that would make me totally dependent on others. I now live successfully alone."

- Death and abandonment in later years.

Increased Disability and Loss of Independence

Poor health and the fear of increased disability are high on the list of significant worries.

Some survivors feel increased weakness in their arms, which may be from using assistive devices that put strain on the joints and muscles over the years. They fear that they will lose the use of their arms, and what areas of their daily life that will affect, e.g., dressing, eating, writing. Others are concerned about loss of mobility, i.e., the inability to walk.

People ask: Can these losses be prevented? Will I be able to continue to be independent? That is where a good physical therapist comes in; one who understands PPS. A physical therapist can teach you how to lessen strain on specific parts of your body. At the same time you learn which muscles to strengthen and how to use them. It is a balancing act, but one that can help you to be mobile and functional.

What is important is knowing when to rest, which usually means trusting your body when it tells you it is tired, and knowing when and how to do activities of daily living.

It may be hard to think about using assistive devices or a wheelchair for getting around. Even getting a handicapped sticker for your car can seem like a big deal, particularly if you have never thought of yourself as disabled. But such aids, once you get used to them, can actually save unwanted stress and strain on your body...and on your mind as well.

PLANNING

To take some of the stress out of life plan for the future, as much as you can. No one wants to think of themselves as needing care or aging—let alone dying, so even thinking of such plans can be stressful in itself.

However, it is not too early to think about what you might do. Be flexible. Don't feel that a plan cannot be changed; that it is written in stone. But knowing that you have a plan can give you some sense of security. You can't cover all bases to be sure, but you can get information and put some plans into action.

Start investigating what your community has to offer. See what others have done. Talk with friends, family, those in your PPS support group. Help arrange a support group meeting where the issues of concern are discussed.

Think realistically about family and friends who would be there for you in a pinch. Some people are very busy, but when push comes to shove they will be there when you need them, and gratefully so.

Housing

You may have thought of moving to a different house or to a different state in your retirement, but are finding the cost of housing prohibitive. If that has happened to you, see how you can arrange your home, where you are currently living.

In wanting to maintain your independence you can start by modifying your home or apartment for easier living now. You might install a few nice-looking grab bars, perhaps a ramp. (Check your town's ordinances about ramps to make sure you are within code and meet ADA standards, if required.) Get rid of nonessential furniture and rugs, so you won't trip or limit your movement in a wheelchair. These are just a few of the things you can do to make your life easier now and in the future.

However, staying in your own home may not be forever. As one gets older and weaker, it is not as easy to maintain your own place, particularly a house. Fixing things yourself may become quite a chore. However, finding a suitable place to live when you are retired, such as a complex with an accessible pool, takes a lot of investigation. More and more retirement villages and apartments are being developed with the needs of senior citizens in mind. It does take some mental adjustments in your self-image to start considering such living quarters. But we all do get older and need to consider the future—as hard as that may be to think about.

Cognitive Therapy Exercises: If you approach these plans early on, when you are not in crisis mode, then you can turn them into interesting investigations. They will not be stressful, but will be a way to see new places and learn new things. Do what you can to see this as an adventure, not a drag. Take pride and relax, knowing that you are doing what you can to take care of yourself.

Financial Concerns

Related to the housing issues are financial concerns. People worry about having financial security throughout their lives. The question I hear is: "Will I have enough money to live on when I retire." You can certainly do some estimates of your assets and income that can help you to live within your means.

Some people consult with a financial advisor. If this is too costly for you, a bank or senior citizens center may be able to refer you to someone. Another possibility is to have the PPS support group get a financial consultant to speak to the group. You can learn something there, and perhaps the group can arrange for an affordable consultation for those who attend the presentation.

HANDLING ANNOYANCES

Remind yourself that life is short and that you have to keep things in perspective. Some of your anger towards annoying situations or irritating people may really be anger at yourself and your situation. Try not to obsess about what bothers you. Don't go over and over it in your mind, or dwell on it when talking to others.

Practice addressing your frustrations and concerns in as mild a manner as you can. That may mean leaving the discussion to another day when you are not so heated up about it. Look for solutions rather than looking for someone to blame. Realize that there is more than one way of doing things. Look for alternatives. Try new approaches.

MANAGING STRESS

One of the first things you can do is to make a list of all the stressful situations you can think of. Don't edit them at first. Just let your mind go and write down as many as you can. Then prioritize the list. Which items are more immediate; which more upsetting, which are more in your control? Group them accordingly with headings.

This may seem like busy work, but actually the act of writing helps you to get away from broad generalizations and overused words that mean nothing specific to you and lead you nowhere.

Now, edit your items. Avoid generalities. Be as concrete as possible. Words mean different things to different people. What do these words mean to you? What does *upset* or *annoy* mean; what does *sad* or *anxious* mean to you?

Take a microscope to each item on the list to see if you can make it very real to you. Ask yourself:

"What's causing the feelings I'm having?"

"Am I feeling overwhelmed, frustrated, out of control?"

Look at your negative thoughts and try to change them to positive ones. On a sheet of paper write down your negative thoughts, such as, "There is nothing I can do." Then beside it in the next column, change this negative thought into a positive one—even something as mild as, "There should be something I can do."

Think of new solutions; let yourself go. Be creative. Say to yourself: "I could do it this way; but what other ways could I approach this? What haven't I done that I could do? Whom can I call? What can I read? Whom can I talk to? What resources are out there? If I am feeling that I must do something, do I really have to do it: Is there someone who could help me?"

Blaming others for problems is very common. It is an outwardly directed, rather than inwardly directed way of dealing with anger and frustration. When things are out of control in your life, looking to authority figures for help is a natural reaction. But when these people let you down, anger can surface.

Communicate

Communication is a very important part of managing stress. One of the ways to find solutions to what troubles you is to *talk* with others and be sure to *listen* to others. But listening doesn't mean that you have to do what others suggest; it is a way of gathering information that you will consider. You may feel comforted to know that others have had to deal with the same issues, and you may learn about their solutions to these problems.

Don't be afraid to ask questions. That is one way to learn. If you are going to a doctor or other professional, you may want to write down your questions, as mentioned in the chapter on working as a team with your doctor. Writing down what you wish to discuss helps you to focus, in case you are a bit anxious. Having the questions in front of you helps you to remember what you want to cover.

Remember that professionals have a limited amount of time, so be sure to edit your questions, and limit them, saving the least important to another time. You may even want to give the doctor your list of questions, letting him/her know that you do not expect all of them to be answered right now, if time is short.

Be Active and Social

Stay as physically active and healthy as you can. Do things to take your mind off your worries. Remember, social support is great for your physical and mental health. So try not to be too much of a hermit. Although interpersonal interactions can be stressful at times, they can also be rewarding. Join a post-polio support group, if there is one in your area. Attend and be active, if you can.

Table 9

WHAT MAKES LIFE STRESSFUL: AN OVERVIEW

GOOD STRESS AND BAD STRESS

Good stress is when we feel we can do something.
Bad stress is when we feel we have no control.

IDENTIFY WHAT STRESSES YOU

Make a list: Write down any problems.
   Don't edit until you have written everything down.

Stay away from generalities. Ask:
   What about this that upsets me?
   What emotions do I feel?
      Worried, anxious, angry, scared, annoyed.

What causes these feelings?
   Lack of control: Can't do anything about it.
   Blocked, frustrated.
   Don't know what to do.

Table 10

MANAGING YOUR STRESS: AN OVERVIEW

THINK OF NEW SOLUTIONS:
Let your mind flow—don't obsess.

STOP NEGATIVE THINKING:
Change negative thoughts to positive ones.
Avoid blaming self or others.
Avoid seeing everything as black.

COMMUNICATE:
Listen to others.
Don't be afraid to ask for or seek help,
e. g., family, friends, doctors, psychologist or other mental health provider, religious counselor.
Don't be afraid to ask questions.

TAKE CARE OF YOUR HEALTH AND BE ACTIVE:
Do things to take your mind off of what troubles you.
Join a support group.

22

TAKING CHARGE OF YOUR LIFE

How do you deal with those parts of your self that you would like to change? For a starter, to make changes in your life—in the way you feel about yourself and in the way you live—you must want to change. Once you make that decision, then you are on your way to asking the important question:

How can I take charge and make changes in my life?

As you learn to identify and understand your anxieties, fear and depression, you then have the opportunity to change how you think and react to events. Thus, no matter what your age, it is always possible to make some modifications in who you are and who you want to be. There are of course limitations.

Our personalities and behaviors can cause us to do things that are either helpful or harmful to our well-being. If you understand your personality, you can make it work for you in more positive ways.

GUIDELINES FOR POSITIVE CHANGE

1. Become aware of how polio affected you as a child and throughout your life.

   Allow yourself to recognize what you went through. Think about what you did as a child to survive polio and its aftermath. Don't expect yourself to have acted or felt as you might now that you are mature. Think about children you know who are the age that you were when you had polio. See how they respond and see the world. You don't expect them to act like adults. So when you look back on your own life, try to understand it through the eyes of the child.

2. Be with others; don't give in to isolation.

   Don't spend too much time alone. Keep active, intellectually and socially. If you get an invitation, consider accepting it. Although it may be easier in the short run to turn it down, that will only lead to more isolation and depression. Be with others. Share their lives and let them share yours.

3. Learn to know who you are, to accept who you are.

   Remember, you can't change your history but you can change the way you re-experience it. You will have reactions to your life experiences, but by:

   a) knowing where these feelings come from,

   b) talking about what you remember, and

   c) talking about what you feel,

   you can help yourself gain understanding and control over your life. Talking out loud and hearing what you say is quite a different experience than just going over and over things in your head.

4. Learn to live with your feelings without letting them run your life.

   If bad feelings come back, try not to act on them. Know what triggers them and try to avoid getting into such negative states or situations.

5. Minimize stress.

   Exercise to whatever extent you can. Get enough sleep, keep caffeine and alcohol intake to a minimum.

6. Look back on events in your life and look for new meanings.

   Tell yourself that you are OK. Focus on your accomplishments. Although you may have an obvious disability, remember that others have their trials and tribulations too; you may just not be able to see them. If you accept yourself and learn to like yourself more, you will convey this to others, and they will act in kind.

23

THE ROLE OF PSYCHOTHERAPY, COUNSELING, AND SUPPORT GROUPS

WHY THERAPY?

On day I received a message on my voice mail from a polio survivor. She had heard that I worked with polio survivors and had wanted to call me for some time—for years in fact, but had been putting it off. She wanted a consultation but ended the message by saying that she was frightened, scared. But what was she afraid of? What was she looking for?

When we finally met, she said she was not sure what she wanted or expected, but somewhere deep inside she was afraid that she would bring up issues and past experiences that she had been unable to face for so long. Would she cry without stopping, scream, shake, and lose control? She did not know. She was afraid of this new venture, which might open up areas that had not been opened up before.

Speaking to a trained mental health profession gives you a safe place in which to work on these troubling issues. You can let things come out slowly, in a manner that is comfortable for you, so that you do not become overwhelmed.

Yet some people feel they need a little push—that left to their own devises they would not go as far as they might like. This is where a trained therapist is very important. One needs to stay within the "comfort level" of the patient.

Others come for a consultation or for several sessions of psychotherapy hoping that the therapist will give them something. They are not sure what they are looking for, but they are searching for something—a "magic bullet" perhaps?

Therapy is not like what you see in a Hollywood movie, where the patient has a dramatic enlightening experience, and then everything is fine afterwards. There is no magic bullet.

Psychotherapy is a journey, an exploration, and one needs to take this journey carefully, learning when to stop and rest, when to go on, and when to step back. That is where the therapist helps you.

Therapy can be a bit one-sided, at least in terms of talking. In traditional psychodynamic therapy, patients do most of the talking—about their past and current life, experiences, and feelings. At first just talking—with what seems like little input from the therapist—makes some patients question if this is worth it.

Rather than giving specific information, often what the therapist does is to provide a framework that leads people to find their own way, to gain an understanding of their life and their emotions, particularly as it relates to their polio experience. They also gain a better understanding of others in their life, both past and present—and learn how to have more control in what seems like uncontrollable situations. Sometimes this means finding new directions to go in or new ways to relate to others.

Over time patients internalize the therapist's voice and way of asking questions. They are then able, when on their own, to ask themselves the questions that will help them find their way.

PSYCHOTHERAPY AND THE POLIO SURVIVOR

Polio survivors can be ambivalent about psychotherapy, wondering how it could possibly help them. However, they may also be avoiding talking about earlier experiences with polio—fearing this will be painful and unleash uncontrollable emotions.

Each person has his or her own reasons for coming to a therapist, and has his or her own individual experiences. People may have feelings that they do not wish to share with family or friends; they may need a place to cry, to complain, and to be understood.

Often those with post-polio syndrome feel that others cannot fully appreciate their distress or cannot abide their need to talk about their difficulties. When they come into therapy, they say they want someone outside of the circle of family and friends to talk to.

Memories from the earlier years with polio begin to surface when the symptoms of post-polio syndrome (PPS) first appear. These memories and associated feelings from the past can lead to generalized anxiety, depression and anger. Through psychological counseling and therapy people gain an understanding of the basis of these feelings and learn how to manage them.

COUNSELING AND PSYCHOTHERPY: SIMILARITIES AND DIFFERENCES

As practiced there can be a lot of overlap between counseling and psychotherapy. Individual counseling and psychotherapy can help people learn to:

- change negative thinking into positive thoughts and actions,
- reduce stress and manage anxiety,
- adopt more effective problem-solving behaviors,
- face the uncertain future,
- improve interpersonal relationships.

Counseling usually focuses on more short-term practical issues and may be helpful you are looking for advice and guidance. Today there is also a new approach similar to counseling, called coaching. Here there is a defined problem and structured ways to deal with the problem and to achieve goals that you set for your life.

Counseling can be more interactive than psychotherapy. In some cases, survivors use counseling to look at new ways to improve their social lives and to make vocational choices. Some work out the issues related to retirement that may come earlier than expected as a result of PPS.

Psychotherapy, particularly what is called psychodynamic psychotherapy, is a more insight-oriented approach and is usually more intense than counseling. This approach is helpful in understanding psychological conflicts from both the past and present. However, it often takes place on a more frequent basis than counseling and over a longer period of time.

When problems make you feel very bad or have been with you for a long time, you may want to consider the kind of help that will get to the root of the problem. Advice and guidance through counseling may not be enough. After a while you are back to feeling the same way, doing the same things and the problems just don't go away. By getting to the root of the problem through psychotherapy, you gain insight into your motivations, and you are able to make changes in your life, in your behavior or in your personality.

For polio survivors, it depends upon the problems that you are dealing with whether you choose psychotherapy or counseling. If you need to make some concrete decisions about well-defined areas in your life, like work or relationships, counseling may be of help. If you are dealing with anxiety and fears of the future or find you want to delve more deeply into how you feel about having polio and what happened to you in the past, then psychotherapy would probably be the best choice. Sometimes a therapist will combine both approaches, counseling and psychotherapy.

In Summary

It is important to point out that going for psychological counseling or therapy does not mean that a person is weak or "crazy." In fact, it is strength to know when to ask for assistance and how to find the appropriate person to help you.

What is most important is to find someone who is qualified and well trained in psychology, psychiatry or social work. That person can help you sort out which approach is good for you. And most likely the therapist will use an eclectic approach, that is a variety of techniques as appropriate.

OTHER FORMS OF TREATMENT

Psychological Techniques:

In addition to "talk-therapy," psychotherapists may draw upon other psychological techniques, depending upon your issues.

Following is a selected description of some of the more common techniques used in Cognitive and Behavioral Therapy.

Behavioral Modification: Rehearsing desired behavior through role playing and establishing new behaviors and goals.

Cognitive Therapy Techniques: Focus on identifying and correcting distorted thinking, controlling unwanted thoughts and behaviors, and developing alternative behaviors or strategies for coping. Some cognitive exercises have been suggested throughout this book. Following are brief overviews of some of the techniques and exercises:

Relaxation Exercises: To help with stress, sleeping difficulties and unwanted thoughts.

- *Imagery*—mentally putting oneself in peaceful situations and focusing ones senses on the details of the scene, e.g., the warmth of the sun on your cheek, the sound of the sea at a beach.

- *Progressive Muscle Relaxation*—concentrating on specific muscle groups, tightening them, then relaxing them, gradually moving from one part of the body to another, i.e., starting with the feet and working up to the head. The intent is to produce a subjective state of calm.

Cognitive Restructuring: Reframing thoughts from those that are negative and defeatist to those that are positive and achievable.

Thought Stopping: Repeating words or phrases over and over to yourself in order to interfere with thoughts that you would like to go away.

Psychiatry and Medication

If talking over your problems does not seem to work for you, then you may want to consult a psychopharmacologist (usually a psychiatrist) to start you on medications to control your depression or anxiety, for example.

Should you decide to take medication, you need to follow what the psychiatrist recommends, and not change dosages or start and stop on your own. Everyone's body is different and some medications work for one and not for another. The doctor needs to follow your treatment and modify what he/she gives you based on how your react to the medication.

There are a lot of new medications out there, without the disturbing side effects of 20 years ago. Some people have found them to be quite helpful, regulating their mood, such as not being so irritable, anxious or sad, and helping them to sleep. In some cases taking medication can speed up the psychotherapy process, as a depression lifts or is controlled, and one has more energy and insight into one's problems.

Family Therapy

As the name implies, family therapy is when members of the family get together with a therapist to improve communication and to work out problems that have developed between couples and within the family system. The therapist facilitates the interchange. This form of therapy can be particularly useful when PPS is involved. It provides a place to work through the changing of roles and the difficulty family members may be having in accepting what is happening.

Family therapy or couples therapy may also be an adjunct to other treatment and can play a psycho-educational role in the lives of the survivors and their families. Coming together to talk about stressors and new adjustments can increase the family's overall ability to communicate and express feelings and needs. This reduces the chaos in the functions of the family, as members learn how to deal with others' fears and gain an understanding of what is going on. Through psychotherapy both the polio survivor and the family members learn to integrate their new and ever changing roles into their lives.

Group Therapy

Group therapy involves a group of people usually with the same or similar issues who come together to help each other gain a better understanding of themselves and how they relate to others. Most often there is a therapist in the room to guide the interchange and to make psychological interpretations, when necessary.

Some people are not comfortable in a group and others just prefer to do things on their own. However, there are those who find group therapy to be helpful and want the input from others.

Group therapy used to be very popular many years ago. It is still available but to a much more limited extent. What has taken its place are "support groups," which are more like counseling in that people share feelings and information, but there is much less of the in-depth analysis of what and why you are doing what you do. Such support groups are usually more educational.

POST-POLIO SUPPORT GROUPS

PPS support groups are not like the old therapy groups of the past, where people came and put all their issues on the table for discussion and analysis by others. Although support group members do share their trials and tribulations, today's support groups have become psycho-social-educational networks, most with their own web sites, newsletters, periodic meetings, and annual conferences with invited speakers.

Post-polio support groups are good for learning about others' coping strategies and for keeping aware of new treatments and specialists. For some, being in a group and learning that others experience the same problems is reassuring. However, for some, a support group may actually increase anxiety, particularly if it means going to a meeting where others with disabilities will be present. Those who previously had milder cases of polio often avoid the group experience at first, particularly if those in the group have obvious and more severe disabilities than they do. Many of these persons have difficulty identifying as "handicapped" or "disabled" and in some cases, seeing persons with more complications makes them anxious about their own eventual prognosis.

It is common for those who have never been to a post-polio meeting to feel anxious about going. Yet once there many have reported that they are energized by the positive and "fighting" attitudes of those they have met and have learned to see themselves in new and positive ways.

For survivors who are unable or unwilling to attend meetings, the newsletters and web sites provide information about PPS—e.g., good doctors, coping strategies, others' histories, research, and new techniques and aids.

Volunteers run most if not all of the post-polio support groups. They dedicate their time and talents, while also trying to live their own lives, and sometimes ask a small fee to cover expenses.

A list of support groups can be obtained from the national organization Post-Polio Health International (formerly G.I.N.I.—See References and Resources at end of this book.)

24

SURVIVING IN UNSETTLING TIMES

With the world experiencing a sense of insecurity, many people for the first time are beginning to know what it means to feel vulnerable. But for those with disabilities, an underlying sense of vulnerability, of a potential lack of control, is not a new experience.

For those with post-polio syndrome (PPS) a sense of vulnerability may have its roots in the early experience with polio, when all of a sudden they could not walk or run, or could not breathe. For the young ones, being sent away by parents to the care of strangers left children feeling unprotected at an age when they were learning how to negotiate and trust in an uncertain world.

GAINING CONTROL

Yet, as we know, most of those with polio made it through those difficult times, and many grew up to be active participants in society, helping to shape the disability movement that has given support to their special needs. By gaining recognition and having these needs met, such as accessibility and equal opportunity, those with disabilities gained more control over their lives and felt less vulnerable.

CONFRONTING NEW THREATS

Then came September 11th and subsequent natural disasters leaving polio survivors wondering: "How safe am I now?" The question is even more poignant for those with mobility problems who, in thinking of escape, wonder how they might survive such disasters.

Yet these incidences revealed that we all have resources we may not know we have. True, some disabled people did perish, but so did many able bodied people. We live our lives knowing that there are risks, but survival comes from remaining strong and vigilant, and working together as part of a larger concerned community.

COPING WITH A SENSE OF VULNERABILITY

From direct experience or watching disasters on television, many people find themselves having difficulty sleeping, or being irritable, anxious, depressed or angry. Those who are experiencing stress from the recent devastating events, may find cognitive techniques useful in helping them cope with these uncertain times.

Talk to others. Remember, you are not alone. Family and friends may be able to reassure you. Those in PPS support groups may share your anxieties and offer useful suggestions for coping.

Be as active as you can. Release physical tension by developing a routine of exercise; even mild exercise is good. For mental stress, relaxation exercises, such as those found on tapes, can be useful.

Reduce the amount of time you spend worrying about things you cannot control or change. Remember that disasters are beyond your control. You can do some planning, but you can't prevent everything. Try to focus your attention on positive images, such as those of people helping others. Help other people yourself, when you can.

Have some modest plans. Although it is hard to plan for the unknown, maintain awareness of whom you can call for help, and keep phone numbers handy. Pay attention to who is around you and where exits are. Even a modest simple plan gives you some sense of control in your life.

Use drugs and alcohol in moderation. They only remove stress temporarily. Limit your intake of caffeine and nicotine, which create stress-like reactions in your body making it harder for you to feel in control. But if your doctor suggests taking anti-anxiety or anti-depressant medication, don't immediately brush it off as the doctor's thinking things are just in your head. Sometimes medication is in order. Talk with your doctor to get more information or get a second opinion.

Consult a professional, if necessary. It is amazing how much stigma there still is in today's world about seeking professional help for your mental health. But if you find that you are spending too much time worrying about life and feeling vulnerable, if you are experiencing thoughts of hopelessness or extreme anger, seek professional help from a certified counselor, social worker, psychologist, or a psychiatrist.

We are all learning to live in these uncertain times.

AFTERWORD:
FACING THE FUTURE

PPS OVER TIME

When I first began working with polio survivors—more than 25 years ago, they would come for psychotherapy to gain an understanding of what was happening to them. Each person's struggle was different, but there were underlying similarities. In many cases they had been developing symptoms of post-polio syndrome (PPS) that lead to unwanted memories intruding into their everyday lives. Some were having difficulties adjusting to new limitations in life style, and others were having feelings that they did not understand: fear, anger, and lack of trust.

Such issues still persist, but with time factors of midlife began imposing themselves as well: Relationship issues with children and spouses, resentments for having to do so much, and upsetting feelings when having one's needs minimized or dismissed.

In time there were also the issues of aging parents, and the conflicting feelings about having to take care of them at a time when post-polio syndrome (PPS) was limiting one's own stamina and function.

With increasing age, additional pressures surfaced: The need to modify one's home or workspace; the resistance to seeing oneself as disabled; and the advent of declining health.

As Karl, a 70-year-old retired mechanic told me:

*"Up to now I could walk. It was very hard but I did it.
I don't want hard anymore."*

TODAY IS THE FUTURE

And now I see a new stage, one that is centered upon the future—a future that is close at hand—not the future of youth, that is so far out there you can put off thinking about tomorrow—but a future that has arrived.

Upon being allowed to stay up past midnight on Christmas Eve, a little boy exclaimed:

"Today is tomorrow!"

And in the tomorrow that is today—with polio survivors in or entering into their later years—new questions emerge:

- How to lead a meaningful life?
- How to make the most of what lies ahead?
- How to prepare oneself for a future that is coming at a galloping speed?

With PPS being full of surprises, it is hard to plan. As one patient described his experience:

*"It's like guerilla warfare.
You never know when, where, or how it will strike next."*

LOOKING FOR ANSWERS

In our culture, where people are living longer, what were traditional roles are not well spelled out anymore. One has to carve out a place for oneself, and this may come at a time when you are having difficulty mustering enough strength just to get going every day.

Allow yourself time to think. To think about what you are doing, what resources you have—financial, health, educational, practical skills.

What would you like to do? If you are able, sign up for one of the courses or vacations that you used to think about taking. Help yourself get over the feeling that you must do something big. That puts much too much pressure on you. Try to be realistic. If just resting and doing nothing but getting through the day is what you have the strength for, then so be it. Accept that and try to make your days as smooth as you can. You have spent a life doing, doing, and doing.

But one needs to be practical too. As much as you may not want to be one of those people who thinks of money all the time, managing your finances is important in our society. There are a lot of holes in our safety nets. Identify how you would want to live, for example, and if you can't afford that, then investigate what resources there may be for you through the government and the community.

If you must scale down your dreams, then now is the time to be realistic and see how to do so. Although you don't want to think about the worse case scenarios, it is not a bad idea to have some plans ready. Worrying only keeps you going in circles. Throughout this book I stress planning. I suggest writing down your thoughts, needs, solutions, and your plans. Writing makes things concrete, so you can really look at what you are thinking, so you can focus your thoughts and your actions.

If you can stay productive in helping others or if you have some interest or talent in the arts, for example, then you stand a chance of feeling some purpose. You may not be able to do what you once did, but you can do something that makes you feel useful, creative, and good about yourself.

SOCIETY TODAY

One last note: Polio survivors have expressed concern about society's lack of attention to people with disabilities. Although progress has been made over the years, those with disabilities face frustrating situations every day.

The progress that has been made in society did not come about by itself. Individuals worked hard to draw attention to the requirements of those with special needs. Individuals fought to get laws changed and barriers removed. Eventually attitudes changed over time as well, but not without the persistent efforts of individuals doing what they could. Each person can make a difference.

You too can make a difference—for yourself, as well as for others.

ABOUT THE AUTHOR

Margaret E. Backman, Ph.D. is a Clinical Psychologist working in the area of Health Psychology. Dr. Backman specializes in helping individuals and families cope with medical illnesses and physical disabilities: She has been working with polio survivors for over 20 years. She has also written numerous articles and given presentations at polio support group meetings and conferences about the psychosocial aspects of the late effects of polio.

Her previous books are:

The Psychology of the Physically Ill Patient: A Clinician's Guide (New York: Plenum Press/Kluver/Springer 1989), *and*

Coping with Choosing a Therapist: A Young Person's Guide to Counseling and Psychotherapy (New York: Rosen 1994).

Dr. Backman is a graduate of Barnard College and received her Ph.D. in Psychological Measurement from Columbia University. She also pursued post-doctoral studies in Clinical Psychology at New York University and completed a post-doctoral fellowship in Cancer Rehabilitation at the Rusk Institute at the New York University Medical School. Dr. Backman has a private practice in New York City.

ON WRITING THE BOOK:
A PERSONAL NOTE

People often ask how I got into working with polio survivors. The other question sometimes asked or at least wondered about is did I ever have polio?

The answer to the second question is: "No, I did not have polio…at least not to my knowledge." As we know, many people had mild cases of polio that were not diagnosed as such, with parents and physicians thinking the symptoms were the flu or something of that sort. But I did grow up during the epidemics of the 1940s and 1950s and was well aware of the threat. Polio was in the psyche and thoughts of everyone.

But how did I get into working with "polios"—as some polio survivors call themselves today? For many years I was the Research Director in a rehabilitation center, to be specific an agency in New York City now called the ICD International Center for the Disabled. I was the project director for the development of the MicroTOWER work samples that evaluated the vocational skills of disabled and disadvantaged individuals. Through my work I got to know many who had disabilities, both clients and colleagues.

Later I had a private psychotherapy practice, and because of my interest in Health Psychology I began to receive referrals from colleagues—referrals that included people who had had polio. This was in the early 1980s, when post-polio syndrome (PPS) was beginning to be understood.

I am a good example of why it is important to educate professionals about post-polio syndrome. One polio survivor frequently gave me literature about PPS. I soon recognized the psychological ramifications of having an illness, such as polio, early in life—specifically the repression of traumatic memories and associated feelings that would be revived later with the advent of new symptoms. This lead to my first publication in this area: *"The Post-Polio Patient: Psychological Issues,"* in the Journal of Rehabilitation in 1987. This was followed by presentations at post-polio support groups and conferences, as well as articles in newsletters. In addition my first book, *The Psychology of the Physically Ill Patient: A Clinicians' Guide* (1989), includes a case study of someone with PPS.

The current book, *The Post-Polio Experience*, draws upon my experience working with polio survivors and covers topics that I have addressed over the years—but with a new look, taking into account that the survivors have aged over the 20 plus years that I have been writing and speaking in this field. Although some of the issues are still important, new concerns have arisen. Thus, some of the material remains as before or has been updated; other material is new or looked at from today's perspective.

REFERENCES AND RESOURCES

OTHER BOOKS ON PPS

Bruno, R. L. *The Polio Paradox: Understanding and Treating "Post-Polio Syndrome" and Chronic Fatigue.* New York: Time Warner Book Group, 2002.

Halstead, L. S. (Ed.). *Managing Post-Polio: A Guide To Living Well With Post-Polio.* Washington, DC: NRH Press, 1998.

Maynard, F. M. & Headley, J. L. *Handbook On The Late Effects Of Poliomyelitis For Physicians And Survivors.* St. Louis, MO: Gazette International Networking Institute (GINI), 1999.

Silver, J. Post-Polio Syndrome: *A Guide For Polio Survivors And Their Families.* New Haven: Yale University Press, 2001.

HISTORICAL REFERENCES

Backman, M.E. (1987) The Post-polio Patient: Psychological Issues," *Journal of Rehabilitation,* 53(4), 23–26.

Backman, M.E. *The Psychology of the Physically Ill Patient: A Clinician's Guide, New York*: Plenum Press/Kluver/Springer, 1989.

Genskow, Jack. (1996). Responding to loss: A practical framework. *Polio Network News,* 12(9), 1–2.

Dobkin, A.B. *Ventilators and Inhalation Therapy,* 2nd ed. Boston: Little, Brown, 1972.

Glud, E. & H.T. Blane (1956) Body Image Changes in Patients with Respiratory Poliomyelitis, *The Nervous Child*, 11(2), 25–39.

Prugh, D., & C. Tagiuri (1954) Emotional Aspects of the Respirator Care of Patients with Poliomyelitis, *Psychosomatic Medicine*, 16, 104–128.

Riesman, David. *The Lonely Crowd.* New Haven, Ct.: Yale University Press, 1961, 1989, 2000.

U.S. Department of Health and Human Services, Report of the Surgeon General's Workshop on Children with Handicaps and Their Families (1982). Case example: *The Ventilator-dependent Child*, Washington, DC: DHHS publication #phs-83-50194.

Van Riper, H.E. (1956) The Parent of the Polio Child, The Nervous Child, 11(2), 40–47.

RESOURCES

Post-Polio Health International
        (Formerly G.I.N.I.)
4207 Lindell Boulevard, #110,
St. Louis, MO 63108-2915.
Tel. 314-534-0475,
www.post-polio.org

Note. Contact G.I.N.I. for information on your local post-polio support group.

978-0-595-38639-0
0-595-38639-3

Printed in the United States
54962LVS00002B/151